ADVANCED LEAN

IN HEALTHCARE

CRAIG T. ALBANESE, MD, MBA
DARIN R. AABY, MS
TERRY S. PLATCHEK, MD

ISBN: 1-4961-4189-X
ISBN 13: 978-1-4961-4189-7
Library of Congress Control Number: 2014904306
CreateSpace Independent Publishing Platform
North Charleston, South Carolina

Dedication

For our patients who place in us their sacred trust, and for our colleagues who have dedicated themselves in service to others.

Contents

Acknowledgements

Continuous improvement is a team sport. You try together, you make mistakes together, you learn together. Writing this book was possible only because of the hard work, tireless dedication, and brave leadership of many, many people. With deep gratitude and great respect, we wish to acknowledge those who have guided us on our quest to provide our patients with the best possible care in an environment that respects and supports those providers who have dedicated their lives to taking care of others.

We are grateful to the executive team at Stanford Children's Health, led by President and CEO Christopher Dawes, and the hospital's board of directors for their recognition that we must confer highest possible value to our pediatric patients and expectant mothers. Our leadership team continues to provide the critical support and resources essential for our lean journey. Our former board chair, John Lillie, who was a very early adopter of lean for commercial transportation, is to be commended for "keeping us honest" and ensuring that we were tenacious in our implementation of a robust management system.

A special thanks needs to be conferred to the brave vanguard of "implementers" at our hospital: Mike Spencer and the performance improvement team, Matt Wolden, Dr. Paul Sharek, and the Center for Quality and Clinical Effectiveness team, and our colleagues in our Perioperative Services department who readily accepted the daunting task of becoming the health system's first model line, Dr. Daniel Murphy who is leading the charge in changing the physicians' view of outpatient care delivery in our organization, and the scores of highly engaged clinicians and ancillary services personnel from pharmacy to maternity and neonatal care and from engineering to information services to acute care—your dedication to our patients warms our hearts and encourages us to continue to improve.

Stanford Children's Health has been fortunate to have partnered with Joan Wellman and Associates from the inception of its lean journey. We are indebted to Joan Wellman and all of her extremely talented colleagues. They asked us to dream about "what could be" and have given us the tools to start us on our journey. Your feedback has been essential to this manuscript. In particular, we have come to realize how fortunate we are to have had access to a Toyota-nurtured sensei, Matt Wehr.

We have been fortunate to have many mentors, teachers, and friends we have met along our journey. Thank you to Colin Fox, former VP of the Terex Business System, from whom we shamelessly stole the hockey to ballet metaphor and for his expert review of this manuscript. Thank you also to our teachers and colleagues who have contributed so much to our professional development as systems improvers. Denise Bennett, Dr. Jack Billi, Dr. Arnie Milstein, Marc Onetto, John Shook, Brad Toussaint, Dr. John Toussaint, and Dr. James Womack, we are in your debt.

So many others contribute to the ever-growing lean knowledge base through a variety of national and international networks and societies. Those most instrumental in allowing us to vet our work and refine our ideas were the Lean Enterprise Institute, the Association for Manufacturing Excellence, the Healthcare Value Network, the Institute for Healthcare Improvement, and the Australasian Lean Healthcare Network.

Thank you to Joni Sensel for helping us clearly articulate our thoughts on the printed page, and to Createspace Publishing (an Amazon company), which exemplifies all of the traits of a very professional, just-in-time, lean company.

Finally, thank you to all of our dear friends, family members, loved ones, and colleagues who have endured endless discussions about "the book." Your encouragement, feedback, and support are gifts for which we will be forever grateful.

Preface

Society's healthcare system needs to deliver reliable quality, safer care, and faster access, all at a lower cost. Many books have been written about the potential for lean management principles to improve the delivery of healthcare services. Although lean management is intuitive in theory, any practical transformation is a long and invariably difficult journey. The goal of this book is to describe a systematic approach that can ease this journey and help you deliver the highest quality, fastest service, and lowest possible cost in the healthcare environment.

The source of this system is not novel. In fact, some readers may scoff at the suggestion that lean management principles can deliver these results, as attempts to implement them in healthcare have met with variable levels of success. Before you make up your mind about it, consider the fundamental principles of a lean operating system:

1. Creates a foundation of stable processes
2. Delivers service just in time, with no customers waiting
3. Delivers perfect quality, with no defects passed on to the customer
4. Ensures the lowest cost possible through employee-led continuous improvement

It is hard to argue that these principles aren't "true north" statements, results that every business should aspire to deliver, so why haven't lean implementations always delivered these results?

The answer lies in how advanced the organization's lean operating system is. Does the organization have a progressive system for developing its people, culture, and management behaviors so that all processes continuously improve with a singular focus on creating value for its customers (patients)? This book explains the maturity levels of a lean system, describing what needs to be in place at each level of the transformation and the returns that can be expected. Most importantly, this book details the progressive steps that drive an advanced lean implementation. Your organization can use these steps to achieve a mature, successful lean system and achieve its mission.

To understand our approach, you must understand our backgrounds. We work on transforming healthcare systems into lean operations while managing them on a daily basis. Our reality consists of engaging executives, clinicians, and staff in lean transformation work while simultaneously trying to give patients high-quality service in systems that are far from perfect. We deal with staffing shortages, patient census shifts, uninterested clinicians, disconnected administrators, broken administrative processes, healthcare reform, and other real-world problems. To face these challenges, we have developed a pragmatic approach to implementing a high-functioning lean system for healthcare environments.

The approach is presented sequentially, building from initial levels to advanced levels. This information is supplemented with practical implementation knowledge and real examples. This book is not an introductory or conversational guide to lean healthcare, and we do not focus on any singular element of lean management (such as 5S—efficient workplace organization) or singular aspect of healthcare (such as outpatient clinics). Rather, we take a holistic and practical approach. Our goal is to provide readers with a framework for progressively implementing an advanced lean system in any healthcare environment.

Executives may ask, "How do we create a high-quality, safe, affordable, continuously improving, proactive healthcare organization worthy of the staff members who have dedicated their lives to serving patients and worthy of the patients who place their sacred trust in that system?" This book answers that question.

CHAPTER 1

From Hockey to Ballet

It's a Monday morning in August, and while most children are enjoying the final weeks of their summer break, an eight-year-old boy named Johnny is waking up in a hospital bed. He has been battling cancer for many months, his disease has progressed, and there is no hope for a cure. After several gut-wrenching discussions with his family, his doctors are transitioning him to hospice care. He is nearing the end of a week-long hospital stay that began with uncertainty over whether he would survive. As fortune would have it, Johnny's condition has stabilized over the past week, and during morning rounds, the medical team determines that he is ready for transfer to an inpatient facility specializing in pediatric hospice care. The plan is to discharge him on Tuesday at 11:00 a.m. The medical team plans to update the family on Monday afternoon.

Like many plans made in hospitals, however, the valiant efforts of caring providers are thwarted by poorly functioning systems, so things don't go according to plan. Johnny's mother arrives at the hospital around noon, about an hour after the team has completed its morning rounds. The medical team, made aware of her arrival, plans to update her in her native language (Spanish) at 3:00 p.m.

Johnny's mother has two concerns she wants addressed. At the time of his admission, it was noted that Johnny's feeding tube (a gastrostomy tube or G-tube) was leaking. Dealing with this issue was deferred because of more pressing concerns, but Johnny's mother wants to address the leak. Generally, this problem is resolved by placing a tube of a slightly larger diameter, which takes only a few minutes.

The second issue is that Johnny's home feeding formula was changed to an inpatient formula during his stay, and his mother wants to switch back to his regular formula when he is discharged, which she notes that he tolerated better.

Given these issues, she raises her concern that a discharge at 11:00 a.m. on Tuesday might be too early. The team agrees, so his discharge is rescheduled for 1:00 p.m., and the case manager starts reworking tasks to reflect the new target.

To address the G-tube leak, those on the medical team need to consult with their gastroenterology colleagues. By 3:30 p.m., they know that a nonurgent consult won't happen until the next day, so they decide to wait to order that consult until Tuesday morning. At the end of the day on Monday, despite the complexity of the discharge, the team feels confident that everything will proceed smoothly.

The next day, however, multiple unintended and unforeseen issues plague the discharge process. In the hospital environment, where both the optimal care of a patient and the care providers can change rapidly and frequently, many physicians learn that it is best to put off writing prescriptions until just before a patient is discharged. This reduces the likelihood that a prescription will need to be changed after it is written, saves time, from the resident's point of view, and sometimes saves rework for the pharmacy. The problem is that last-minute prescriptions often delay patient discharges.

Johnny's case is no different. After the team rounds on Johnny at 10:00 a.m. on Tuesday, they begin preparing his prescriptions. Using the electronic health record (EHR), it takes forty-five minutes to reconcile his thirteen medications (a process that clinicians often describe as frustrating). The physician sends the prescriptions to the printer. The printer is out of prescription paper, resulting in a ten-minute search for the correct paper. Worse still, when the paper is found, the physician needs to reprint each prescription individually, because the electronic ordering system allows batch printing only on the first attempt. The medication orders are brought to the outpatient pharmacy at 12:15 p.m. It is obvious that a 1:00 p.m. discharge will not happen, and the case manager works to notify everyone involved of the delay.

As the pharmacy tries to fill the prescriptions, it notes that a particular medication is not available. Over the next several hours, multiple attempts at communication are made between the pharmacist and the attending physician, who is in the clinic. Processing for all the prescriptions is put on hold while waiting to clarify the medication in question.

While this saga is unfolding, the gastroenterology team adjusts its schedule to see Johnny in an expedited fashion. After its consultation at 12:30 p.m., it notes an issue: the hospital doesn't stock the G-tube in the size that Johnny needs. Several calls are made to find a hospital-associated vendor who can courier the tube to the hospital that afternoon, but Johnny's discharge time must be changed twice more. Due to unclear communication, a clerk in the vendor's office calls Johnny's mother to ask if the G-tube order is correct. Thinking that the hospital (not the vendor) will provide the tube, Johnny's mother cancels the order. The case manager catches the error but not before another ninety-minute delay and the need to complete yet another new order.

Over the next several hours, the discharge target is changed three times, and each instance requires the case manager to update the palliative care facility and the transportation team. By 4:00 p.m., Johnny's home-feeding formula has been sorted out, and he has his G-tube replaced. He has his medications in hand, although the labels, originally printed in Spanish, must be quickly reprinted in English and Spanish because he has multiple caregivers.

As the transport team prepares Johnny for transport, it notices that a "Do Not Resuscitate" order has not been signed. This physician order, which is appropriate for Johnny's care, instructs the paramedics not to attempt resuscitation if Johnny's breathing or heart should stop during transport. No one can find a blank form.

While the search ensues, the receiving institution calls, asking for a summary note of the patient's stay. This note, which can take over an hour to write, is normally completed within twenty-four hours of discharge, but because Johnny is transferring facilities, it needs to be completed prior to his discharge. The team simply forgot.

At 4:45 p.m., after a mad rush of paperwork and four missed discharge times, Johnny leaves the hospital to take what is likely his last car ride.

We can only hope that the night team at the palliative care facility, now tasked with Johnny's admission, has a more reliable process.

This poorly executed discharge not only affected Johnny and his family, but it diverted the attention of staff, physicians, and management from other patients for an unnecessarily long time. It is not hard to imagine the quality or safety implications for other patients on the unit, not to mention the staff dissatisfaction, with this type of work. We can also imagine the frustration that Johnny's mother must have felt as her faith in the system dwindled with every misstep, particularly when facing an emotional tidal wave and knowing that her child has an imminently fatal condition.

While certain facts have been changed to protect patient identity, this is a true story recorded by the performance improvement team at our hospital. It represents an all-too-common scenario in hospitals across America—one in which patients and their families suffer under systems of care that don't perform to expectations.

Still worse is the fact that to many clinicians, this story might not seem so bad. After all, Johnny wasn't administered an incorrect medication, and he didn't contract a hospital-acquired infection. This may be "business as usual" to many clinicians. In fact, in most hospitals, Johnny's case would likely be noted as a routine discharge that happened in the late afternoon; the administration would be blissfully unaware that anything unexpected or out of sorts had happened. The cumulative impact of work-arounds, inefficiencies, and missteps is mostly hidden from doctors', nurses' and hospital managers' collective views but not, of course, from our patients. In addition, this type of mayhem is an underlying theme that contributes to healthcare worker burnout.

Herein lies our great challenge: How do we get the entire healthcare system to start paying attention to inadequate care processes and management? Does the process have to seriously harm a patient to get our attention? If we wait for serious harm or financial Armageddon before we pay attention to our systems, we will continue to fail! We contend that preventable mistakes such as these lead to poor-quality care and preventable harm.

Johnny and his family got lucky in that he wasn't harmed. He *was* at risk, as were the other patients on his ward who were ignored because of the chaos that his discharge created.

A Fresh Approach

After many years of work in the American healthcare system, it has become evident to the authors that doing the right thing by our patients is much more difficult than it should be. "Healthcare exceptionalism"—the belief that healthcare provision is so unique, complicated, challenging, and regulated that any lessons to be learned from other industries are largely irrelevant—is prevalent in healthcare leadership. The familiar refrain exempting healthcare from the market pressures faced by other industries is becoming deafening; it might be comical if it wasn't so serious. Close to one out of every five dollars spent in the United States is spent on healthcare. Healthcare can no longer be exempt from finding ways to reduce unnecessary variability, simplify systems, cross-train and fully use the talents of workers, and warranty services. Is the $8,500 colonoscopy in one city demonstrably better than the one in another city for $1,900? Probably not.

The idea that our healthcare system could provide higher quality and more compassionate care, at lower cost, stands in opposition to the notion of healthcare exceptionalism. Under the premise of exceptionalism, every stakeholder in the system becomes logically constrained by the belief that no improvement can be made without substantially increasing resources. Consequently, the reality has become that staff, clinicians, and patients are forced to navigate an overly complex, inefficient, and service-unfriendly environment.

In this book, we use an analogy that we hope resonates with you. Present-day healthcare is much like an ice hockey match, while our proposed state, created using systematic lean principles, looks much more like ballet.

Despite planning, practice, and preparation, a hockey game is fundamentally unpredictable; no one can say where the puck will be ten minutes into the match. We are not suggesting that hockey is a haphazard sport. Quite the opposite; hockey players hone their skills to take variability out of the game by controlling the puck. In contrast, ballet artists know the next move before it happens, so there is no need to react quickly to an unknown input.

In Mike Rother's book[1] about people development at Toyota, he describes the systems and skills needed to produce precisely choreographed patterns for work processes and performance improvement. He likens these movements to those seen in Japanese Kabuki, karate, and the tea ceremony. Despite the immense training and preparation of its workforce, healthcare is largely based on aligning resources around unpredictable patients and variable care pathways, analogous to hockey. To turn healthcare into ballet, the bulk of the variability must be taken out of the system so that staff members can follow a set routine, regardless of a patient's clinical condition.

Understanding Patient Variability

We acknowledge that patient populations are incredibly diverse and variable. In addition, the complexity and chronicity of diseases increase as innovative medical treatments and long-term care progress. However, our experience has taught us that the variability in healthcare is due to an unstable operating system and lack of clinical standardized work (i.e., care pathways) that is rigorously followed for all patient populations—simple and complex, acute and chronic. Much of the variability we see as healthcare workers is self-imposed.

It is our responsibility to care for the increasingly complex cases and the chronically ill patients in the system, but it is also our responsibility to minimize the complexity of daily healthcare operations. Healthcare can no longer tolerate unnecessary, costly operational complexity. For example, before our process improvement work began, the operating rooms in our hospital had the following problems:

- Much of the requisite preoperative paperwork was completed late, usually on the day of the surgery.
- Many patients arrived late.
- The schedule of cases was determined by physicians based on their personal views of what constituted optimal patient flow within their blocks. This was done with no regard to overall recovery room capacity and demand or intake unit workflow.
- The recovery room was staffed according to historical data, not actual caseloads.
- Patients developed unexpected clinical events, such as an unexpected prolongation of a procedure in the operating room.

These variations can be separated into three groups:

1. Demand. Inputs into the system (patients) arrive at varying and often unpredictable times. (This corresponds to the patients arriving late and a physician-determined schedule in the aforementioned bulleted points.)
2. Operational. Processes are completed (or not) without a clearly articulated and followed standardized method. (This corresponds to incomplete paperwork and historical staffing.)

3. Clinical. Patients fail to follow the expected clinical course. (This corresponds to an unexpected prolongation of the surgical procedure due to an unexpected clinical event)

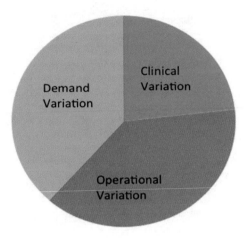

Figure 1.1: Types of variability in healthcare

In our experience, demand and operational variation account for the largest proportion of variability (Figure 1.1)—both in the aforementioned operating room example and in the healthcare system overall. This variation leads to staff and patient dissatisfaction as well as work that is unsafe and costly. Fortunately, unlike unexpected clinical variation, demand and operational variation are often in our control, particularly operational variation. These variations can be minimized by eliminating wasteful processes and standardizing work (these concepts are discussed later).

Unfortunately, unless the variation is studied carefully, we tend to be biased by anecdotal cases of clinical variation. This bias is often generalized with statements such as "Patient care cannot be timed, scheduled, and made to follow standard guidelines. Patients are simply too variable—they are not like cars on an assembly line."

This myth can be debunked by creating a stable system. Otherwise, a state like a hockey game will persist; well-intentioned, well-trained people will react to the unpredictable ricochet of the puck. Those striving to score will miss the net, others will miss passes, and others will skate to the puck only to find it quickly sent in another direction. All variations that can happen will do so relatively consistently. This is a good thing for the game of hockey—it's what makes it a terrifically exciting sport, but it is not how we should care for patients.

To exemplify this further, consider airport operations. To move to a state of a well-choreographed and predictable "ballet," a plane needs to safely land at regular times. Like healthcare, the airplane faces demand variation (variability in the number of planes wanting to land at a given time), operational variation (variability in the work that the ground crew is performing), and environmental variation (unforeseen variability in flight times due to uncontrollable factors like weather, which is akin to clinical patient variation). All these factors degrade an airport's ability to safely land the maximum number of planes in a given day (Figure 1.2). Over time, however, airport managers learn to deal with these variations so they can act more like a ballet troupe than a hockey team.

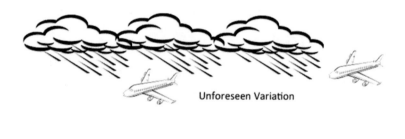

Unforeseen Variation

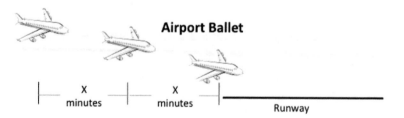

Airport Ballet

Figure 1.2: Airports maintain steady flow with unforeseen variation

As shown in figure 1.3, modern airports have air traffic controllers, flight scheduling teams, pilots, and ground crews all working together to maintain a cadence. This is how they ensure on-time flights more than 80 percent of the time despite the inherent, unexpected variation in air travel. This performance is astounding, given the potential and actual variation in the aviation industry.

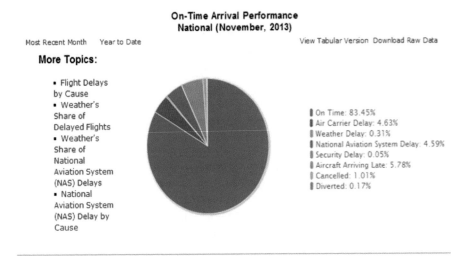

On-Time Arrival Performance
National (November, 2013)

Most Recent Month   Year to Date   View Tabular Version Download Raw Data

More Topics:

• Flight Delays by Cause
• Weather's Share of Delayed Flights
• Weather's Share of National Aviation System (NAS) Delays
• National Aviation System (NAS) Delay by Cause

▌On Time: 83.45%
▌Air Carrier Delay: 4.63%
▌Weather Delay: 0.31%
▌National Aviation System Delay: 4.59%
▌Security Delay: 0.05%
▌Aircraft Arriving Late: 5.78%
▌Cancelled: 1.01%
▌Diverted: 0.17%

A flight is considered delayed when it arrived 15 or more minutes than the schedule (see definitions in Frequently Asked Questions). Delayed minutes are calculated for delayed flights only.
When multiple causes are assigned to one delayed flight, each cause is prorated based on delayed minutes it is responsible for. The displayed numbers are rounded and may not add up to the total.

Figure 1.3: Causes of variation at airports

To make ballet possible in healthcare, it is critical to set up systems that allow patients' clinical conditions to vary while ensuring stable on-time operations. It is important to recognize that not all variation needs to be removed to make significant progress. Just as ballet dancers get better with practice, the performance of a healthcare organization will improve as variation is removed.

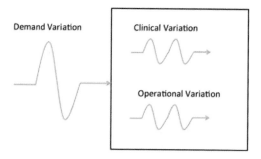

Figure 1.4a: Current state = hockey

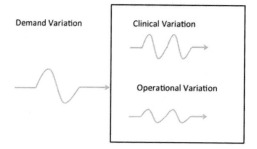

Figure 1.4b: Starting ballet

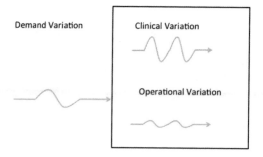

Figure 1.4c: Better ballet

As shown in figures 1.4a–c, the only variation line not progressively dampened is the one depicting clinical variation. We leave clinical variation in a class of uncontrollable circumstances, (similar to poor weather for airplanes that will need to be dealt with) and recognize that it is difficult to eliminate. Thus, our mantra is "let clinical variation be the only variation that exists in the healthcare system."

Smoothing Patient Flow

The patient flow diagram in figure 1.5 was modeled from our operating rooms (ORs) before we implemented an advanced operating system. It shows how unpredictable and variable workloads were on a given day; several surges of patients were followed by times with virtually no patient work for the staff and clinicians.

Current Healthcare System (Hockey)

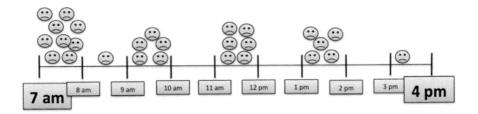

Figure 1.5: Unleveled patient flow

As noted earlier, this variability and unpredictability created a system that was unreasonable for workers. High-stress, "get 'em through" periods were followed by periods of "not a lot to do, we had better look busy." In addition to adversely impacting the staff, this workflow increased costs and reduced quality for patients. Unpredictability is acceptable in hockey, because the goal of the game is to be variable and exciting. Unpredictability is not acceptable in health-care, however, because our goal is to treat patients consistently and reliably. We submit that the tenets of a well-choreographed ballet are a far better model for healthcare: be reliable, consistent, and predictable. By using a variety of lean principles, we can distribute patient flow and staff work more evenly through-out the day (Figure 1.6).

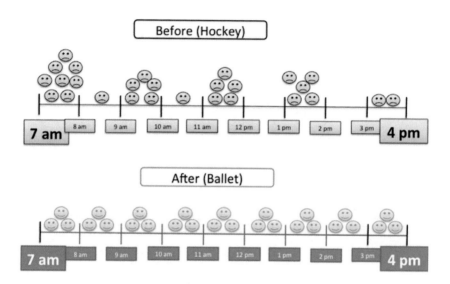

Figure 1.6: Unleveled vs. Leveled patient flow

Our approach to moving from hockey to ballet can be described in five levels. (See chapter 4 for details.) Most of these levels should not be new to students of lean management in healthcare. What is paramount is that the major trans-formation—what we call the "advanced lean system" (i.e., moving from hockey to ballet)—requires creating a system built around a consistent work cadence or tempo in response to *patient* needs. The tempo should be smooth and generally predictable, even if variable. Just as the precise choreography of ballet is the basis of its beauty, a well-choreographed patient flow that eliminates ebbs and surges can serve as the basis for a care system that is reasonable for both patients and providers.

Focusing on the Principles

You may find yourself questioning the sense of trying to equate healthcare with ballet. After all, healthcare is more like hockey—patients, like pucks, are less than 100 percent predictable. The delivery of patient care does not seem particularly analogous to assembly-line work, so how can these concepts translate to healthcare? The answer lies in understanding the principles of ballet and not focusing on specific solutions. Although there will be a multitude of solutions to achieve ballet in healthcare, only three principles need to be met.

Principle 1: Match capacity to demand. Always match capacity (the workers' ability to serve) to demand (the patients' need for service). Historically, lean operations have addressed this principle by leveling demand and serving a consistent number of patients per hour, which allows for level capacity (e.g., consistent work hours for staff). The value of stabilizing working hours makes leveling demand the preferred method when possible. What if demand (patient flow) cannot be leveled? In this case, staff will need to be moved flexibly in and out of areas as patient demand dictates. In practice, we find that most areas employ a combination of leveling demand and flexible staffing to match capacity to demand. It should be noted that in the current state, few healthcare organizations can detect real-time demand swings throughout the organization, let alone flex resources to the areas where they are needed most.

Principle 2: No waiting. Patients deserve service without undue waiting. When processes get behind, it takes heroics by the staff to get the processes back on track to serve the growing patient queue. Unstable operating systems often deliver unforeseen problems (e.g., uneven scheduling) that force staff members to improvise and patients to wait. These conditions exemplify the conditions of hockey that must be eliminated if we are to truly have ballet in healthcare. In addition, the organization needs a mechanism that keeps staff on track in real time. In this system, management's primary job is to keep each area on track by applying the necessary resources, in real time, to eliminate unnecessary patient waiting.

Principle 3: Perfect quality. We must ensure that poor quality and safety errors will not be passed on to patients. This requires a mechanism to stop and fix issues as they occur. At first glance, this might seem like a nice idea that works for other industries but can't be employed in healthcare. Would we ask a patient's progression through the system to stop while a quality issue is fixed? We believe that the answer must be a resounding "Yes!" From sponges left inside patients to treatment halts due to incorrect paperwork or not properly washing hands before contacting a patient—all quality and safety issues must be identified and dealt with immediately if we are to have choreographed care delivery—ballet. Linking quality and safety in a "stop-and-fix" manner puts quality correctly ahead of efficiency. Staff members are not allowed to move on to other patients if they still have a quality or safety issue to address with the current patient.

These principles will be discussed in detail in later chapters, but a specific example on how they can be applied to the highly dynamic world of healthcare follows. The chart below (Figure 1.7) presents an example of patient flow into an actual emergency department (ED), with a lot of demand variability in patient arrivals per hour. On Monday through Thursday, the shape of the demand curve from day to day is virtually identical.

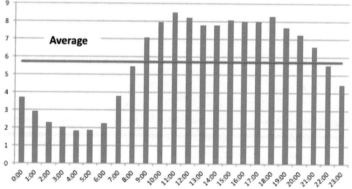

Figure 1.7: ED hourly demand curve

Knowing this repeatable variability, the ED team could take the following measures:

1. Match the staffing plan to the repeatable daily demand curve. In this case, at 11:00 p.m., the ED needs approximately four times as many resources as at 5:00 a.m. (Principle 1: Match capacity to demand).
2. Implement a management function that monitors patient flow in real time and can move resources in and out of the ED as needed (Principle 1: Match capacity to demand).
3. Change management's focus to keep staff on track and operating at their expected rate (Principle 2: No waiting).
4. Employ a "stop-and-fix" method to all quality and safety issues (Principle 3: Perfect quality).

In step 4, clinicians and area management focus on serving patients at an expected rate with perfect quality. If patient care takes longer than expected, it is management's job to understand why and immediately fix issues under the staff's control so that other patients don't suffer undue waiting. If a patient's clinical condition requires more than the expected time, so be it—uncontrollable clinical variation has occurred.

The key at this point is not to get too involved with the specifics of how to create ballet in a given area; the later chapters address implementing ballet in specific areas. For now, we hope that the principles of leveling to demand, no waiting, and perfect quality give a sense of our method.

Here is a brief overview of the steps to transform healthcare from hockey (controlled chaos) to ballet (choreography).

1. **Create an aligned organization.** Develop and communicate an organizational vision for aligning around quality, the patient and staff experience, and patient flow. At this juncture, nothing will have changed in the work areas; this is the time for setting a vision of what healthcare ballet will look like in practice.

2. **Create operational stability.** Here the focus needs to be on creating reliable work processes so that staff and clinicians have what they need when they need it. Establish reliable access to equipment, supplies, and information, and ensure that reasonable staffing plans exist. Although nothing has been done yet to smooth patient flow (i.e., you are still playing hockey), these changes will make real improvements to the workflow of the staff and clinicians. The work at this step is analogous to setting the stage for ballet but still playing hockey albeit with better equipment or smoother ice. This is an absolute precondition for moving from hockey to ballet.

3. **Align by value stream (patient flow), establish a cadence, and match capacity to demand.** Now that work areas are operationally stable, it is time to move to the first step in the transformation. This is done by clearly defining the set of processes—called a value stream— that are involved in meeting patient needs. With a value stream flow, all processes are set up around a horizontal patient flow, not a clinician flow (also called vertical or siloed flow). (See Figure 1.8 for this horizontal approach, which is discussed in chapter 3.) With the value stream in clear relief, we must understand the overall patient demand, determine the cadence of that demand, and, wherever possible, flow patients through the system at that cadence. The work at this step is analogous to writing a script and setting the tempo—it is the first stage of ballet.

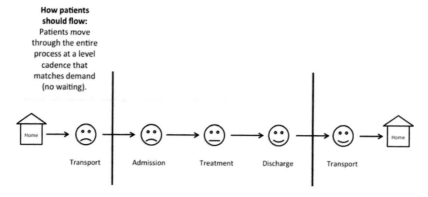

Figure 1.8: Value stream flow = patient flow

Once flow is established for a value stream, leveling the workload is essential. As patient demand and staff capacity become more matched, work increasingly progresses at the cadence that matches patient demand. This allows staff to be efficient while patients receive care in a "no-wait" environment.

4. **Design and implement consistent standardized work for staff and clinicians.** This step requires the staff to perform their work methods in an allotted time so that they can reliably respond to the established patient cadence of demand. (This patient cadence of demand, called "takt time," will be explained in chapters 4 and 8.) This will be done by designing the work methods with the staff and clinicians who perform the work on a daily basis, not simply with area management. The goal is to create reliable staff and clinician work capacity so that it can be matched to the leveled patient flow. This work, which is analogous to choreographing the cast (staff, clinicians, and management), denotes further progression of the ballet.

It is essential that all work sequences have built-in mechanisms aimed at ensuring perfect quality. They should prompt and empower frontline workers (nurses, physicians, and other direct patient-care professionals) to stop and fix issues (process stop) before errors are passed along in the system, thus preventing harm to patients. Because management's chief responsibility is to maintain patient flow (progression), if there is a process stop (e.g., a patient's care cannot progress due to a quality issue), management's job is to respond immediately and help fix the issue so that patient flow can resume (Figure 1.9). Moreover, it is critical to find and fix the cause of the problem so it never happens again, thereby decreasing the likelihood of a process stop in the future. With this mindset, the frontline staff's job is to stop patient progression when a quality or safety issue is identified, and the managers' job is to resolve the issue quickly so that the patient journey can resume.

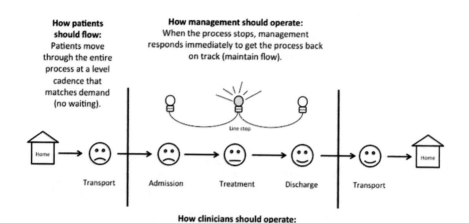

How patients should flow: Patients move through the entire process at a level cadence that matches demand (no waiting).

How management should operate: When the process stops, management responds immediately to get the process back on track (maintain flow).

Line stop

Home → Transport → Admission → Treatment → Discharge → Transport → Home

How clinicians should operate: Error proofing is built into all work sequences. If work sequences cannot be completed in the planned cycle time (i.e., perform just -in-time service with perfect quality), clinicians stop the process.

Figure 1.9: Process stop ensures quality

5. **Continuously improve the performance (for better ballet).** Once consistent work methods for staff and clinicians have been established and the system is performing to the established cadence, we can move into the final phase: continuously improving flow by challenging the system to further improve the work standards. This is achieved using the methods (steps 1–4 above) used to get to this stage, eliminating the issues that are causing the patient flow to stop. Management, staff, and clinicians conduct daily process improvements aimed at preventing process stop conditions from recurring (Figure 1.10). These improvements are integrated into the daily standardized work, where use proves whether or not they are actual improvements. This scientifically based improvement cycle—Plan, Do, Check, Adjust (PDCA)—has no end. As staff members become proficient at hitting their allotted work sequence times, management works with them to further lower the allotted time (creating a new standard) so that process stops and daily PDCA are required to meet the new standard.

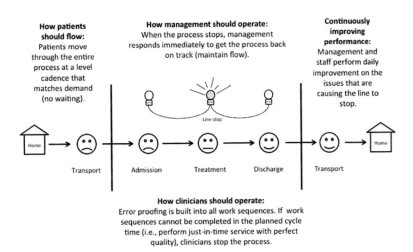

Figure 1.10: Continuous improvement ensures better and better performance

This system can be depicted by a five-tiered "house" that largely replicates the Toyota Production System house (Figure 1.11). However, the "advanced lean healthcare house" (further described in chapter 4) depicts the natural upward progression, via the five levels, of using the tools required to produce the "true north" outputs at the top of the house. The patient-centric, waste-elimination system creates healthcare of the highest empathy and quality, lowest cost, and fastest delivery.

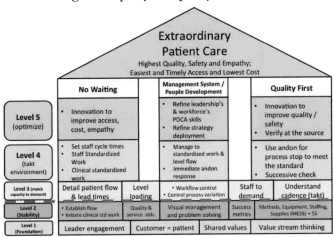

Figure 1.11: Advanced lean healthcare operating system

Our definition of advanced (versus basic) lies in an organization's ability to move past the red line from levels 1 and 2 (hockey) to levels 3 through 5 (ballet). Though this is a relatively systematic, multilevel approach, it has nuances that require in-depth discussion, particularly around developing a daily management system/people (culture) and the oft-noted seesaw pattern of implementation among levels. As you read the subsequent chapters, ask yourself how an advanced lean operating system, if in place and functioning well, would change the care experience for Johnny, his family, and the staff caring for him.

CHAPTER 2

Defining Value

In 2014, healthcare reform is taking shape in the United States. It is clear that the American healthcare industry needs to improve its quality of care, provide that quality without preventable harm, ensure exceptional service to patients, and create an ideal staff experience. These goals must be accomplished with the fewest resources (space, people, and money) possible if there is any hope of achieving sustainable near-universal access to care. Furthermore, the underlying principles for these goals, which are founded on care for an individual, need to be extended across the care continuum to serve diverse patient populations.

In 1999, the Institute of Medicine published its landmark call to action report *To Err is Human: Building a Safer Healthcare System.*[2] The authors, invoking the Hippocratic oath, rightly questioned whether a healthcare system built on the principle "first do no harm" could come to terms with the fact that it was killing as many as ninety-eight thousand people a year in hospitals as a result of preventable medical errors. Since that time, studies have looked at harm in hospitals in a variety of settings.[3,4] These studies noted that harm to patients occurs in an astonishing 25 to 49 percent of hospital admissions, and over half of those incidents can be ascribed to preventable causes. These trends, if unchecked, will continue to undermine the foundation of the healthcare system: the trust that patients place in their providers.

While the epidemic of patient harm continues to plague the healthcare system, costs for healthcare in the United States have surpassed 18 percent of the gross domestic product, and they continue to rise. In an article published in the *Journal of the American Medical Association,* Berwick and Hackbarth estimated that in 2011, failures in healthcare delivery and coordination accounted for over $150 billion in annual costs.[5] They found that overtreatment and administrative complexity accounted for an astronomical $440 billion in wasted annual expenditures. Put in perspective, the combined cost of waste exceeded the 2011 defense budget by over $50 billion and was more than seventeen times the budget of the National Institutes of Health. On a microeconomic level, there may come a day when organizations can charge only $800 for a magnetic resonance image that actually costs $3,000. Over the long term, that kind of a cost differential will destroy an organization's viability. We'll always need capital projects such as new buildings or electronic record systems, which will add to healthcare's already out-of-control operating costs.

Taken together, the issues of errors and runaway costs represent a moral challenge for our healthcare system. No longer can we accept the harm created by how we provide healthcare, and we can't afford to spend our way out of quality problems. Fortunately, there is a way to reduce costs and improve quality at the same time, and it is called lean management or, in shorthand, "lean."

A System to Create Value

To be successful, healthcare enterprises need to deliver on four key elements:

1. Provide patients with the best-known options to improve their health or alleviate their suffering (in other words, "deliver clinical quality").
2. Provide patients an exceptional service experience.
3. Provide empathetic, compassionate care by implementing a system that does not overburden staff and clinicians and that promotes their professional development and sense of mission.
4. Provide services affordably and in a sustainable (profitable) way so that the healthcare enterprise can prosper over the long term.

These four elements form the basis of what a healthcare enterprise is meant to produce. Said another way, *they define how a healthcare organization creates value.* The elements of clinical quality outcomes, patient experiences, staff experiences, and fiscal responsibility (i.e., cost or corporate sustainability) can be represented by the value equation depicted in Figure 2.1.

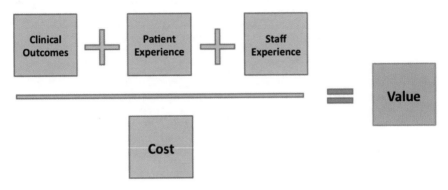

Figure 2.1: Value equation

It becomes easier to think about creating high value in healthcare by defining the four components of the equation as their *ideals.*

1. **Perfect clinical outcomes.** Health is improved and suffering is alleviated, to the limits of medical science, as desired by the patient and without preventable harm.
2. **Ideal patient experience.** Create the optimal healing environment across the continuum of care by providing timely access and minimal waiting for services and by meeting the patients' spiritual and emotional needs.
3. **Ideal staff experience.** Fulfilled staff (both clinical and nonclinical employees) makes for empathetic care providers. Providing a reasonable workload, meaningful work, support by management at all levels, a safe work environment, a culture of respect, and good income/benefits drive the staff experience.

4. **The lowest cost.** Use the minimum resources to efficiently and effectively optimize experiences of the patient and the staff.

The value equation above represents how a healthcare *enterprise* creates value for its patients. We believe that this equation also represents value from the patient's perspective. However, it is often not obvious where or if the "ideal staff experience" fits into the equation given the oft-quoted definitions of valuable service from the patient's perspective:

- Quality/cost
- Something that a patient would pay for (e.g., a patient would not pay for time wasted in a waiting room)
- Outcomes that matter to the patient at an affordable price

Based on these definitions of value, would a patient "pay" for the ideal staff experience? Is an ideal staff experience *necessary* to produce outcomes that matter to the patient? We strongly believe that an ideal staff experience is a prerequisite for high value. It is our experience that a focus on creating the ideal staff experience has been missing from many lean transformations. If the system cannot maximize the time and talent of its workers, the healing environment will be suboptimal. Conversely, a system that creates an ideal staff experience is calm, quiet, relatively predictable, safe (e.g., minimal work days lost due to preventable injury), has minimal absenteeism, and, most importantly, creates *time* for empathetic connections—the human touch. This is what differentiates healthcare from manufacturing. We interact face-to-face with our customers (patients), and they look to us to deliver care physically (through tasks), intellectually (through critical thinking and problem solving) and emotionally (taking the time to listen, educate, and confer compassion). Simply stating that value is, for example, simply quality/cost trivializes the impact of the workforce on patient healing. To maximize value for our patients, we believe that rather than a small improvement to the same old system, a new way of operating—a move from hockey to ballet—is needed.

Value as Described by the Patient: Quality and Safety, First and Foremost

Regardless of whether you are talking about cars, computers, hotels, or healthcare, there is no quicker way to make customers dissatisfied than by asking them pay for something that doesn't work. In their book *The Machine That Changed the World*,[6] Womack, Jones, and Roos described Toyota's managerial system of lean production resulting from the Massachusetts Institute of Technology's five-year study identifying production factors leading to success in the global automobile manufacturing industry. The message of the book was that Toyota found a way to provide much higher-quality cars at a significantly lower cost than its competitors. Toyota's approach is relevant to healthcare because the principles described have little to do with cars and everything to do with how humans create value as a team. Because healthcare has evolved from single providers practicing in isolation to groups of providers practicing as a complex team, we have much to learn from the study of other complex systems.

The first lesson is the most important: quality is king. In the past fifteen years, it has been refreshing to see an increasing emphasis on quality and safety within the healthcare industry. As described in the Institute of Medicine reports *To Err is Human*[2] and *Crossing the Quality Chasm*,[7] the Joint Commission's *National Patient Safety Goals*,[8] and the Institute for Healthcare Improvement's 5 Million Lives campaign,[9] healthcare providers are increasingly aware of the perils associated with the provision of care that's growing in complexity. More healthcare providers will be judged on the quality of care they provide, and we all stand to benefit. When patients place their well-being—in many cases, their lives—in the hands of healthcare professionals, we owe them the highest quality and safest care possible.

The test of successful healthcare organizations in the coming years will be how well they ensure quality. So long as people are involved in a process, errors are guaranteed to happen; the trick is keeping them from reaching the patient. There are common (and expensive) ways of ensuring a high level of quality: increasing the numbers of inspectors and auditors, double and triple checks with multiple providers, countless hours of education and reeducation, and massive over-resourcing. The less expensive ways of ensuring a high level of quality include error-proofing, visual signals, and continuous improvement methods that rely on lean principles.

Value as Defined by the Patient Experience

The most essential objective for any organization is exceeding customer expectations; it is one of the keys to growing a healthy company. Customers are the basis of every business, and if they are not delighted, they "vote with their feet" and go elsewhere to find the services that meet or exceed their needs. Although they want a broad variety of things, basic needs never go out of style, regardless of the industry: high quality, low cost, and easy accessibility. This is as true for customers purchasing bananas as it is for a person getting an annual physical exam.

Figure 2.2 outlines the steps that a customer must complete to buy bananas from a supermarket. It depicts a purchase event characterized by convenience, no waiting, a high-quality product, and competitive cost.

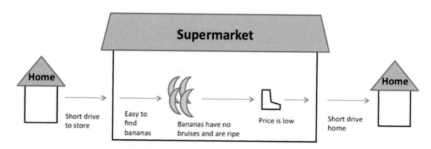

Figure 2.2: Steps required to obtain goods in a supermarket setting

It appears that the price and quality are good, but what about the time and gas spent on the drive to the store? The harder it is for customers to obtain what they want from a particular supplier, the more likely they are to find a different supplier. If they can order bananas online and have them delivered to their house for the same cost and quality, they might switch suppliers. This kind of opportunity must be guarded against to prevent losing otherwise loyal customers. No matter how good they are, businesses must continuously improve their services to ensure that customers continue to receive the highest quality, lowest cost, and most accessible products possible.

Now that we've studied a simple banana purchase, let's shift to the process of getting a physical examination from a clinician, as depicted in figure 2.3:

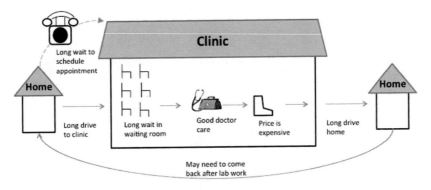

Figure 2.3: Steps required to obtain a service in a healthcare setting

In the example of buying bananas, there aren't many barriers that would drive customers to look for an alternate banana supplier. In the case of this clinic, however, patients face an access barrier (a long wait to schedule the appointment), a long drive to the clinic, and long wait times. Additionally, they may have to repeat the entire cycle if they have to come back after laboratory blood work is complete, sometimes just to be told that everything is normal. There is also a price problem; the service is seen as expensive by the patients (or their insurer or employer). If patients can get the same quality of service in a nearby walk-in clinic with a short wait time, if they know of a clinic that guarantees that the lab work will be done at the same visit, or if they find a clinic that has lower prices, they might switch to those locations.

The importance of high quality, low cost, and high availability cannot be understated. These goals may sound like common sense—and they are! Many healthcare organizations would say that they are already working on many of these goals. Hospital-acquired conditions (i.e. preventable harm), cost reduction, and access are important metrics in most institutions. With the focus on these metrics, aren't we already taking most, if not all, of the right steps to accomplish what patients need?

The simple answer is no. Although many in healthcare share the goal of meeting these metrics, the traditional healthcare model does not have patient flow at the center, which is why the lofty goals of zero preventable harm, no waiting, and low cost cannot begin to be reached.

Figure 2.4 depicts a high-quality encounter at a clinic that has a lean operating system.

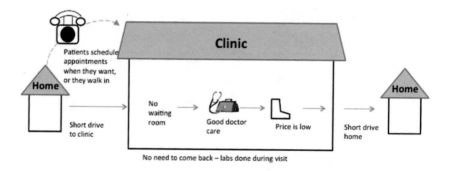

Figure 2.4: Lean model (value stream flow) focuses on
keeping patients flowing with no waiting

From the lean perspective, the experience of receiving a physical examination should be similar to the experience of buying bananas. Patients should expect easy access to quality care at low prices. In an increasingly competitive market, the healthcare institutions that deliver on these goals will take patients from those that do not.

Empathy as a Differentiator for the Customer Experience

Lean was popularized by Toyota Corporation's production of high-quality, low-cost cars in an environment that supported efficient and reasonable staff work. In contrast to the interaction between car parts and the humans assembling those parts, the delivery of healthcare requires direct human-to-human interaction in the "assembly" of direct patient care. Empathy—defined as identification with and understanding of another's situation, feelings, and motives—is key when it comes to delivering a great customer experience.

Research completed at Massachusetts General Hospital and published in the *Journal of General Internal Medicine* in 2012 revealed that empathy in healthcare was essential to the formation of strong patient/physician relationships as well as positive patient outcomes and overall satisfaction with the experience.[10] Empathy is without a doubt a human connection, but in healthcare, it's much more. It's about letting people know that they matter and that clinicians care about their well-being. Clinicians need to connect with their patients on a personal level, treating each one as a person, not as a diagnosis. Listening to the customer's (or patient's) voice is a key tenet of a lean system.

Part of the ideal patient experience is making the healthcare system easy to navigate, minimizing waiting, and delivering the highest-quality clinical care. It is as important, if not more, for clinicians to spend time with their patients, connect on an emotional and/or spiritual level, and encourage them and their families to take part in the decision making for their care. This cannot be done if the day-to-day operations in a healthcare setting are chaotic. Chaos unnecessarily subsumes portions of the staff's and clinician's time—time that could be spent with patients. It is disheartening to recognize that some staff members unknowingly "check their souls" at the front door of the hospital, disheartened by the daily struggles of working in a complex and unpredictable system. Without operational stability and adequate time for patient care, the connections that an empathic healing environment depends on will be hard to create. With a stable operating system, time can be given back to clinicians and their patients.

Pathway to Mutual Prosperity

It cannot be overstated how dependent a lean operating system is on the engagement of *all* the people within it. From executives and managers to physicians, nurses, and other staff, everyone must be involved if the extraordinary gains of the highest levels of empathy and quality, no waiting, and the lowest possible cost are to be realized. Lean is a people-based system that ties everyone's work together to promote the smoothest possible patient flow. If one person doesn't do his or her part, the whole team suffers (not to mention the patient). Disengaged healthcare workers are by far the biggest reason for lean failure.

To get past this hurdle, a mutual prosperity agreement (i.e., if the healthcare worker gains, patients gain) must directly tie quality, cost, access, and empathy for the patient to the concept of "what's in it for me" (WIIFM) for the healthcare worker (Figure 2.5). Although WIIFM will vary from person to person, it can be described by a work environment that provides the following:

1. Meaningful work
2. A reasonable workload
3. Management support at all levels
4. Consistent, good income and benefits
5. A culture of respect, which includes a safe work environment

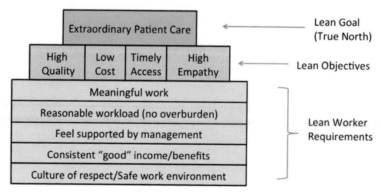

Figure 2.5: Value Proposition "mutual prosperity" between an organization's workers and the patient

Asking workers to work harder, work longer hours, and "firefight" problems as they emerge and reemerge is not a sustainable system. The system needs stability, and this stability must be tied to the mission of the system (also known as "true north"): the satisfied customer or patient. In this system, workers at all levels need to feel undying support from management. People need permission to fail, and management needs to support them when they struggle. This is the most important thing leadership can do to ensure a successful lean transformation.

In this model, senior managers must be present in the workplace and must consistently emphasize that their job is to help overcome barriers for the people who care for patients. Managing from an office or conference room does not work in this system, and that is one of the primary reasons that lean systems stall or fail. (This problem is discussed in chapter 5.)

Respect must be present throughout the workplace. This includes not only respect from the staff, clinicians, and management toward patients and their families but also toward each other. Roles, responsibilities, seniority, personal beliefs, and backgrounds will differ within an organization, but these differences must be embraced and leveraged to build strong teams. Leveraging the collective talent and experience of all workers will also ensure continuous improvement of ourselves, of others, and of the processes that best serve the desired patient outcomes.

The culture must include a strong desire to eliminate preventable harm. This message is often expressed for patient care, but it is vitally important to protect the staff from injuries such as body fluid splashes, needle sticks, and ergonomic and lifting injuries.

It is vitally important that managers develop their people into expert problem solvers, coaches, and future leaders. In this way, succession planning is inherent in the system.

When senior managers are present and supportive, communicate their roles as enablers, deliver on that promise, and reinforce a culture that puts the patient and staff experiences at the heart of quality and value, they set the foundation for a stable operational system. Such a system can muster the resources for improvements (summarized in the next chapter) that enable the staff to deliver superb quality and empathetic care in a timely manner and at a lower cost. Engaged and empathetic staff members who enjoy their work and are mission driven will put the needs of the patients above their own.

Lean as a Stable Operating System: Two Compelling Reasons

Senior healthcare executives must address issues from healthcare reform, accountable care organization (ACO), and electronic health record (EHR) systems to joint ventures and other methods of growth and differentiation. All must be implemented with an eye toward sharing the risks with payers based on the value of service delivered rather than the volume of service. The diversity of elements in a complete healthcare enterprise is represented as items on a platter in figure 2.6.

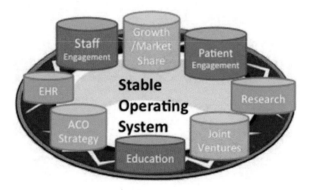

Figure 2.6: A stable operating system supports all the
interests of the enterprise

We submit that these "must do/can't fail" items are more likely to succeed when the organization's operations are stable (predictable and sustainable). If operations are not delivering high-quality outcomes, day-to-day issues quickly consume an organization's resources and ability to do anything else. We have found that many managers can clearly articulate their short- and long-term strategies. Describing the operating system in detail (the "platter") needed to support these strategic goals (the "entrees") is more difficult. Do you have a system (represented by the "?" in Figure 2.7), and if so, what are its components, and how predictable is it? The goal of this book is to help you define and create a stable operational foundation that supports your enterprise's strategic goals.

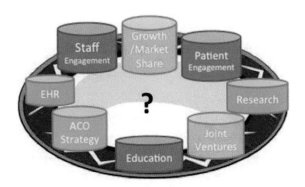

Figure 2.7: What are the key attributes of a stable operating system?

If you are a nonclinical staff member (engineer, materials manager, transport, and their managers) or a clinician (nurse, nurse practitioner, physician assistant, pharmacist, physical or occupational therapist or physician), you have probably been plagued by an uneven workload, a suboptimal work environment, missing supplies, and a lack of timely patient care information. You have probably witnessed preventable quality and safety events. The goal of this book is to help your organization create a stable operating system that will enable you to better support your patients' needs and improve your workplace experience.

Common Organizational Obstacles That Can Impede a Successful Lean Journey

There are many obstacles to a successful lean journey in healthcare. If not recognized and addressed, they can prevent the initiation, slow the transformation, stall the transformation, or lead to complete failure. We will address obstacles such as the differences between manufacturing and healthcare, organization-wide project portfolios, traditional medical education, and the common healthcare organizational structure. Related issues that can impede a lean journey (executive and staff alignment, lean leadership culture, and leadership behaviors) are discussed in chapter 5.

People Are Not Cars

It is no secret that successful and sustainable lean process improvements have been attained in the car manufacturing industry, particularly at Toyota. Are the principles used to improve customer value in car manufacturing germane to an industry that cares for patients? We believe the answer is yes. The examples below illustrate some of the challenges that healthcare organizations must recognize and manage as they begin a lean journey.

All industry sectors have three things in common: inputs, processes, and outputs. In healthcare, the inputs are patients, the processes are the clinical and nonclinical tasks done to support patient care, and the outputs are the measures of the quality of the processes (mortality, morbidity, service standards, cost, to name a few). Lean focuses on improving processes so that any organization, in any sector, can do lean.

As discussed in chapter one, continuous improvement efforts must focus on optimizing the most controllable processes and minimizing input variation. The system can then better manage an unexpected event (such as an assembly-line stoppage due to faulty equipment in a factory or a patient having a severe adverse reaction to a drug in a hospital).

Lean optimization is rooted in rapid and iterative PDCA cycles. This strategy is no different from how a care provider manages a patient's clinical condition: diagnose the condition, plan a treatment, do the treatment, check the results of the treatment, and adjust the treatment if necessary. However, healthcare must also embrace the PDCA concept for solving process problems. Once this concept is embraced and woven into the fabric of the organization, the potential for improving the "health" of the organization is limitless.

Regardless of the industry, creating customer value is the central tenet of a lean operating system. Customer value is achieved by creating a people development-based operating system that enables expert daily problem solving (continuous improvement) through iterative learning (i.e., PDCA) cycles. Lean manufacturing has embraced the concept of "customer first," and it defines the customer as the person who purchases the item the manufacturer produced. Although "customer first" is espoused by many healthcare organizations, in practice, the customer is often viewed as the physician, not the patient—processes are often optimized with respect to *physician flow* rather than *patient flow*. The effect is unsatisfied patients and thus unsatisfied physicians and other healthcare workers. This situation must be changed, and we believe it can be changed.

There is also the issue of mixed product lines. At any time, Toyota may be making cars to meet a variety of customer specifications. Similarly, healthcare organizations care for patients with different needs. The critical differences are complexity and scale. For example, Toyota may have six types of cars on the line at any time. In contrast, a hospital may be treating sixty types of diseases in patients of varying heights, weights, and ages at any time. Although both systems are complex, healthcare is much more complex. This doesn't mean that healthcare can't better manage its processes and clinical care using lean methods; it means that it must do so by understanding the constraints imposed by the expertise required to care for the varied patient populations. For example, every line worker at Toyota is trained to perform four different jobs. In healthcare, medical assistants can be cross-trained for different outpatient clinics, and fewer technicians and nurses can be cross-trained, but it is virtually impossible to make a rheumatologist perform rheumatology care one minute and heart surgery and endoscopic procedures the next.

The key difference between manufacturing and healthcare is that healthcare interfaces directly with its customer, the patient. In manufacturing, customers are unseen to the workers. In healthcare, processes and improvements need to take into account the need to empathetically connect with customers, garner trust, involve patients in their care plans, educate them, and make time for those much-needed human interactions. It is our hope that lean process improvement will give the healthcare system the time and predictability to maximally humanize medicine.

Large Project Portfolios Make It difficult for Executives to See a Lean Transformation as Anything but Another Project

Healthcare organizations need to do more with less. This is why committing to lean as an operating method has been so appealing to so many. Against this reality is a mountain of perceived "must-do" projects that get in the way of spending the necessary time and resources on an enterprise-wide advanced lean transformation. Typical programs that compete for executives' energies are implementing new information technology (IT) systems, building new facilities, negotiating with nursing unions, creating joint ventures, and expanding marketing efforts. Because all of these initiatives are meant to help the organization stay relevant, it makes sense that executives would want to work on them. Because developing a lean operating system doesn't answer all of their concerns, they may have a hard time maintaining their focus on it. If the executive team takes on too many large projects at once, it will overwhelm itself and the organization, which will only make matters worse.

The effective countermeasure is to pick a few (two or three) critical, large-scale projects at the enterprise level, and stick with them until they are complete. In practice, this is difficult to do, because there are always many more than two or three enterprise-level projects that seem critical. The key is to understand the organization's project capacity limitations. This can be done by understanding that typical operational units are staffed only to do their daily work. At best, they will have the capacity for only one enterprise-level project in addition to their daily operations. Once the executive team agrees to this, it becomes clear that the organization's true capacity for enterprise-wide initiatives is typically two to three.

Although the projects that make the "critical few" list is up to each executive team, we suggest viewing your organization's performance through your patient's eyes as the starting point. Ask, "Do we have an operating method that ensures an excellent patient experience and continuously improves?" If the answer is not yes, we strongly suggest picking lean as one of your "critical few" enterprise-wide initiatives.

Formal Healthcare Training (Nursing and Medical Schools) Teaches Good Disease Management but Poor Process Management

Many middle managers in healthcare operations are great clinicians and leaders who rose through the ranks into positions of operational authority. They have been taught from healthcare school onward that the people capable of heroic efforts rise through the ranks the quickest. Unfortunately, this runs counter to what is asked of a lean leader, where diving deep and solving problems at their root replaces a "quick-fix" mentality.

To illustrate, let's use a cardiac surgeon's workflow. When the surgeon fixes a blocked artery in the heart, she is financially rewarded. No one can argue that fixing the blocked artery is of critical importance, but in a way, it is not addressing the root cause of the problem (heart disease). The surgeon repeats the operation and is rewarded each time. It doesn't financially benefit the surgeon to solve the issue with her patient through better diet, exercise, and avoiding smoking and alcohol, all of which could help to prevent heart disease. Instead of fixing the cause of the patient's problems, the healthcare "reward" system is based on endless, complex cycles of rework.

Additionally, the complexity of clinical work makes it hard to address seemingly simple operational process with the necessary amount of humility. Clinicians tend to be humble when it comes to diagnosing and understanding medical issues. The heart surgeon, for example, would never proceed with an operation without confirming catheterization data that supports the diagnosis of coronary artery disease. This is why treatment cannot begin before tests results are received, even when the surgeon thinks she knows what the problem is. Even if she was right 95 percent of the time (that is, 5 percent of the diagnoses were wrong), how many unnecessary operations would that lead to?

A similar approach needs to be employed when designing and implementing operational processes. Until the prevailing attitude is that process problems, similar to clinical problems, are often not easy to fix and comments like "just do what I told you, and that will fix the problem" are heard no more, implementing an advanced lean system in healthcare will not be possible.

Disconnected Reporting Structures Need to Be Dealt With

In most businesses, the reporting structures are clearly aligned around their product (Figure 2.8a). Everyone reports to leaders who eventually report to a central leadership team that oversees the creation of a high-quality product for its customers. This alignment streamlines the organization's ability to focus and make efficient and effective decisions that support customer requirements. In healthcare, this type of alignment does not often exist (Figure 2.8b). Typically, there are at least two different reporting structures: hospital operations and physicians. In teaching institutions, there are more, because the school of medicine adds at least one more reporting structure to the mix.

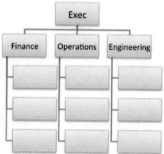

Figure 2.8a: Typical business
alignment

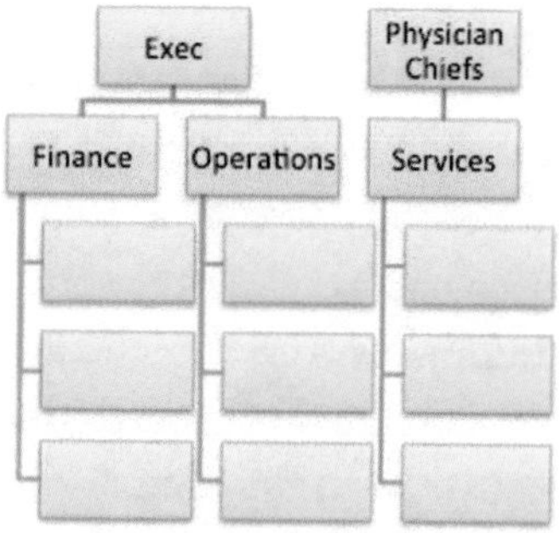

Figure 2.8b: Typical healthcare
alignment

With these disconnected reporting structures, it is difficult to get consensus on what the top two to three enterprise initiatives should be and even harder to get the disconnected groups who report to management engaged. Still, this is the state of healthcare, and so we need to bridge the gaps. Compacts between physicians, the executive team, and the medical school in teaching institutions have proven effective.

The key is to align all teams around the organization's central mission with the patient as the primary customer. Optimally, a compact should be in place before starting a lean transformation initiative so that all groups are on board from the start. Without buy-in from executive stakeholders, an advanced lean transformation cannot be achieved. Like compacts, some institutions have started to compensate parties who are present at lean improvement events or who are working on ongoing lean transformation work in their own areas.

CHAPTER 3

Lean Fundamentals

Because this book focuses on the advanced principles required for a comprehensive, patient-centric system, this chapter presents the fundamentals that are key to understanding the proposed system. It provides a high-level overview of these lean fundamentals: *gemba*, value stream alignment, PDCA, *muda* (waste), *muri* (overburden), *mura* (unevenness), zero defects, and continuous improvement.

Common lean concepts such as *andon, takt,* cycle and lead times, flow, mistake proofing, and standardized work are defined in the appropriate chapters. Common techniques for lean problem-solving—A3 thinking, 5S, process mapping, quality function deployment, 3P (see chapter 9), single piece flow, and hosting improvement events—are covered in the books listed in the bibliography.

Gemba

In lean systems, the Japanese term *gemba* is used to describe the *location* of any step that adds value to the customer—i.e., a step that the customer would be willing to pay for or one that brings the patient closer to the desired outcome. Gemba is easy to identify, because it is always in direct contact with the customer (patient). That's one reason why "going to the gemba and seeing with your own eyes" is stressed when managing lean systems. In the banana example in chapter 2, the gemba is the store, and understanding how easy it is to navigate the store is best done by purchasing bananas yourself.

This approach can be applied in healthcare. Let's use the outpatient clinic as an example. Going to the clinic and experiencing the services yourself is the only way to see how well value is being provided. Charts and graphs in a conference room meeting of leaders will not provide the experience of how well value is conferred to the patients. Issues such as how long patients wait, how many times they have to repeat information, how pleasant the staff is, or how much attention staff members pay to washing their hands before they make contact with the patient are all much clearer when you go through the experience yourself and "walk the gemba." A common lean concept used to describe this experience is "The Three Actuals" rule. Go to the actual place where patients are treated, watch the actual processes being performed, and speak with the actual people doing the work for the patients.

In all healthcare organizations, there should be a tiered accountability mechanism for all processes leading to the desired quality, safety, service, and cost. There should be serial checks of key process and outcome metrics by management and their direct line reports: vice presidents oversee/coach/develop their directors, directors oversee/coach/develop their managers, and so on. While doing these checks, the phrase "going to the gemba" is often misused. For example, a vice president may state that he is going to visit his direct report's "gemba," which does not include direct contact with the patient. Technically speaking, this is not the actual gemba, because it doesn't directly impact the patient's care. It is important to understand that oversight of one's direct reports and going to the true gemba (where patients are receiving care) to learn about the issues impeding patient flow are not mutually exclusive, and *both should be practiced each day*.

Gemba	Not Gemba
A patient calling for an appointment	The clinic manager creating a staffing plan
A physician writing a prescription for a patient	A director auditing a manager's work
Discharging a patient on an inpatient unit	A conference in the executive boardroom

Table 3.1: Gemba defined

The examples in Table 3.1 offer important clues into the thinking behind lean. Because the steps that directly lead to the patient's desired healthcare outcome are value added, all other activities, no matter how necessary, do not add value, and are termed "waste." It's critically important to understand that everything that does not directly affect the patient's progression at the moment the patient is being served is non-value added work. Value added steps exist only where the patient is being directly served in the gemba.

It is also important to string the value added steps together so that the patient experience can be improved throughout the entire encounter. The string of value added steps a given patient goes through for a given treatment, from start to finish, is called the "value stream."

Value Stream Alignment: Shifting Focus from Providers to Patients

How does lean deliver high-quality, timely service at the lowest possible cost, and why is it different from other operating systems? The primary difference is the laser focus on those processes that best serve the patient. It is natural for most businesses to want to optimize the output of whatever they are skilled at. In healthcare, patients seek medical help from physicians, so the natural focus has been on optimizing the healthcare provider's flow, not the patient's. Large waiting rooms and multiple visits might help providers stay busy, but they degrade the patient experience since they add unnecessary cost and waste the patient's time.

This focus on optimizing the flow of healthcare providers is commonly called "siloed" flow, and it is present nearly everywhere in healthcare. From hospital rounds and clinic waiting rooms to batch processing of laboratory tests and routine instruction on managing chronic disease, processes are built around optimizing provider flow. Make no mistake; this does not happen because of selfish intent. Siloed flow optimization happens because it appears to be the most efficient way of doing things when viewed from within the vertical silo (Figure 3.1).

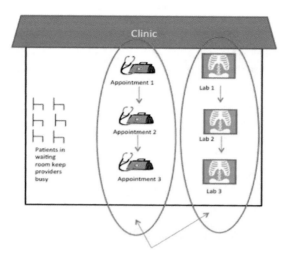

Figure 3.1: The traditional model (siloed flow) focuses on
keeping providers flowing with no waiting

The paradigm shift in lean is to shift the focus from providers to patients.
Focusing on optimizing the flow of patients is commonly called "value stream
flow," and it requires looking horizontally across many silos to see how care can
be optimized (Figure 3.2).

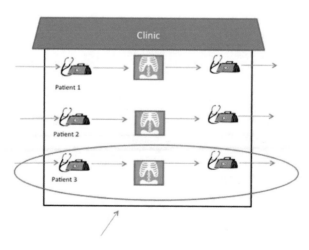

Figure 3.2: The lean model (value stream flow) focuses on
keeping patients flowing with no waiting

Healthcare providers must understand that high quality (that is, healthier patients) alone is not enough; low cost, timely access, and an empathic approach must also be present. Along with high quality comes integration along the continuum of care, depicted as the horizontal oval in figure 3.2. This value stream focus begs the question: Won't the focus on patient flow destroy the efficiencies of the physicians? When lean is done correctly, the answer is no, because low cost is a primary requirement of the patients. If providers are poorly used, their fees must be applied across fewer cases, which raises the cost of a visit to the physician's office. Making physicians and staff more efficient by enabling them to see more patients in a day is a critical requirement of a lean healthcare system.

As a real example that shows how lean can benefit staff, clinicians, and patients, the authors' lean improvement team addressed the labor and delivery operating rooms (ORs) where procedures did not start on time, thereby wasting patient, staff, and clinician time. Once the current state was mapped, the siloed flows became clear. Obstetricians, anesthesiologists, nurses, and technicians all marched to their own drumbeat, optimizing their sub-processes when prepping the patient for the OR. A value steam flow was implemented, linking the work for the obstetrician, anesthesiologist, nurses, and technicians into a continuous patient flow (Figure 3.3) which easily revealed system waste. After the change, on-time OR starts increased 97 percent, thereby eliminating wasted time for patients and providers. This improvement could occur only by aligning the team around horizontal (nonsiloed) patient flow.

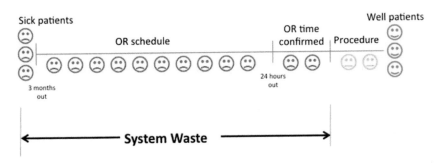

Figure 3.3: Value stream flow reveals the waste from the patient's point of view

Value Added versus Non-Value Added

As stated earlier, all work that goes on throughout the day is divided into two categories: value added and non-value added. The steps that directly lead to the patient's desired healthcare outcome are value added work. Non-value added work (waste) is everything else. Viewed through that lens, only the frontline staff performs value added work, and even then, only a percentage of their time is spent in value added operations. Just because work is non-value added, however, does not mean that it is not necessary. Activities such as quality audits, supply ordering, personnel reviews, or taking out the trash are non-value added but clearly necessary. The objective of lean management is to *eliminate* steps that are both unnecessary and non-value added steps and *minimize* the necessary but non-value added steps through continuous improvement. Figure 3.4 shows how this relationship works.

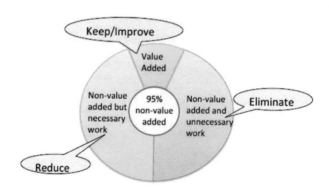

Figure 3.4: Focus on waste

Muda: Waste

Continuous improvement through the elimination of waste is one of the most basic mantras of lean teaching. On the surface, this seems simple: Just fix things, and you are doing lean work. Although there is some validity to this reasoning, the true goal is more specific—namely, making the patient's experience better through eliminating waste (*muda*). Here again, the patient's requirements of low cost, high quality, easy accessibility, and high empathy must come into play when defining where waste exists so that the issues that matter most can be improved.

Historically, waste has been grouped into the eight categories (Table 3.2.) These activities add cost, increase waiting, and/or decrease quality, so they should be targeted early in lean transformation work.

Waste Category	Definition	Healthcare Examples
Correction	Rework because of defects, low quality, errors	• Requisition form incomplete/inaccurate/illegible • Order entry error
Overproduction	Producing more, sooner, or faster than required by the next process	• Unused printed results/reports • Unnecessary labs/visits
Motion	Unnecessary staff movement (travel, searching, walking)	• Walking to and from copier/office/exam room • Searching for misplaced form/equipment/chart
Material Movement	Unnecessary patient or material movement	• Multiple patient/paperwork transfers • Temporary locations for supplies
Waiting	People, machine, and information idle time	• Patient in waiting room • Wait for lab results
Inventory	Information, material, or patient in queue or stock	• Patient waiting in exam room • Excess stored supplies
Processing	Redundant or unnecessary processing	• Reentry of patient demographics • Repeat collection of data
Underutilization	Underutilized abilities of people	• Nurses refilling Rx or making appointments • Physicians doing simple patient education

Table 3.2: Eight types of waste in healthcare

It is interesting thing to note how much waste is present in any system when viewed through the lens of the patient. In Figure 3.5, all the steps required to administer a dose of medication are classified into value added and non-value added, using the definitions provided in table 3.2. (For example, a patient would not pay to wait unnecessarily in a clinic but would pay to be examined by a healthcare provider). In the example in Figure 3.5, 93.6 percent of staff time is used in non-value added activities. This is not unusual in healthcare. The only value added steps are the physician's order, the preparation of the medication by the pharmacist, and the administration of the medication by the nurse.

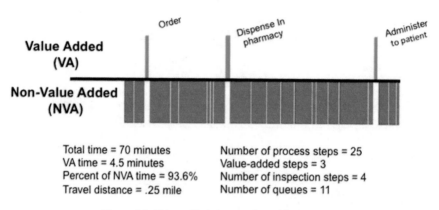

Figure 3.5: Value added / non-value added timeline

This amount of waste is typical; most processes consist of 90–95 percent waste. Because some of the waste is non-value added but necessary, an initial waste-reduction goal of 50 percent would be an excellent target. One of the principle benefits of waste elimination is giving time back to the system. This is time that practitioners can spend making personal connections with their patients, seeing more patients in the clinic, or performing additional procedures in the operating room (or time that non-clinicians can use to keep the environment safe and maximize the support functions for patient care).

As waste-elimination work in an area progresses, the key is to implement work standards so that the staff can repeat the improved methods, thus raising the overall area's efficiency. In addition to codifying "the best way we know how" to do a given job, standards can also be used as powerful continuous improvement mechanisms. One of the founders of the Toyota Production System, Taiichi Ohno, stated, "Without a standard, there can be no improvement." His simple idea is the basis for the scientific method; it is impossible to make lasting improvements to unstable systems.

PDCA: The Core of Continuous Improvement

The cycle of creating standards, implementing them, and continuously improving them is the basis of continuous improvement in a lean system. PDCA outlines the steps that must be completed in one complete improvement cycle. The images in Figure 3.6 below demonstrate Ohno's view that one cannot truly improve a process without first standardizing it.

Let's use figure 3.6 to illustrate a hypothetical target condition of decreasing central venous catheter infections. One of the principle drivers of a central-line infection is the sequence of events necessary for changing the line's dressing. Figure 3.6a shows the impact on the target condition (e.g., fewer infections) if all nurses on a particular unit have their "own" way (i.e. non-standardized process) of dressing a catheter. Hitting the target will be sporadic at best. Once the process is standardized, all nurses are educated to that standard, and as the new standard is monitored, the dots tend to coalesce (Figure 3.6b)). As the standard improves, the unit begins to hit the target and lower the central-line infection rate (Figure 3.6c).

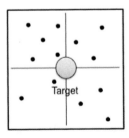
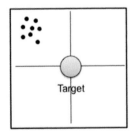
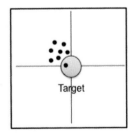

Figure 3.6a: Process with no standard

Figure 3.6b: Process with a standard

Figure 3.6c: Process with an improved standard

Going from the middle box to the right box requires one or more PDCA cycles of problem solving. Each PDCA cycle is supported by a "wedge" or the new standard, shown in figure 3.7. This wedge, which includes attention and support by management, prevents reverting to the old process.

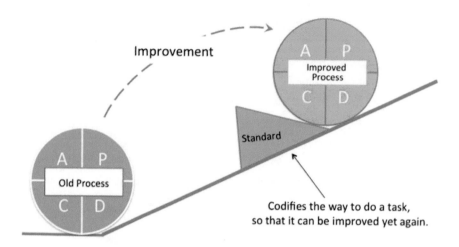

Figure 3.7: Standards hold process improvement gains

It is important to note that standards are not just for the staff and clinicians; all jobs (including those of executives and support services such as human resources and finance) need standardized work so that they can operate with high efficiency and continuously improve.

Taking Entropy into Account

Entropy is a universal law that works to constantly reduce the efficiency of any system. A newly painted house provides an example. When the house is first painted, it looks the best it ever will. As time goes on, the paint will deteriorate until the house needs to be repainted.

Organizational entropy shows up as process improvements that are not sustained (Figure 3.8a). As new, "improved" processes are implemented, we should expect a steady deterioration of performance unless we do something to counteract entropy. This is where management comes in, as it is the managers' job to perform the maintenance needed and keep the standards from suffering from entropy (Figure 3.8b). This constant maintenance is a big change from traditional management, but it needs to be addressed for improved standards to be sustained.

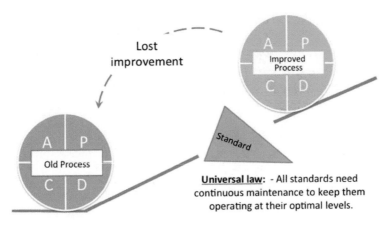

Figure 3.8a: Standards erode over time

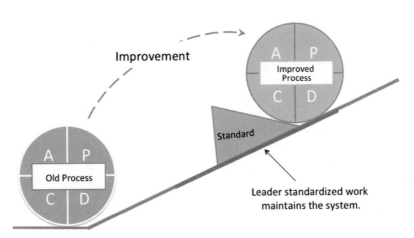

Figure 3.8b: Leader standardized work: Holds process improvement gains by maintaining the standards

Muri: Overburden

Lean calls for appealing outcomes: continuous improvement, mentoring and coaching at all levels, perfect quality, and high efficiency. These ideals, and the hope for a better healthcare system, can galvanize people around implementing lean systems for their daily work. However, without a workplace that can support spending time to work on lean each day, all transformation efforts will eventually wither and die. People need consistent time and opportunity to focus on a lean transformation. Unfortunately, the healthcare work environment allows precious little time to do more than "fight fires" while caring for patients.

If we are going to transform the work environment from the game of hockey to the art of ballet, we need to allow the proper time and make training available to the entire healthcare team. If we can't, improvement efforts will be like giving players better hockey sticks or smoothing the ice—making the game better in small increments but not resulting in the more predictable flow and reasonable tempo that would characterize ballet. If we do a good job at eliminating waste and leveling the workload, a reasonable work environment, with minimal overloading (*muri*), will result.

Mura: Unevenness

To understand the concept of mura, conduct this experiment. Fill a large cup with water. You have five minutes to drink the water. Drink at a steady pace—not too slow, not too fast—so that the cup is empty in exactly five minutes. Fill the cup again. You have five minutes to drink the water, but this time start the clock, wait thirty seconds, and drink half the water in one second. Wait for the clock to read 4:59, and in the last second, drink the other half of the water.

The same amount of fluid will be consumed in the same amount of time, but the experience will be different. It's obvious that slow and steady is a much better way to drink than gulping and waiting. Gulping large volumes in a short time creates problems: running out of breath, spitting, and possibly choking. In addition, waiting between gulps is boring and is inefficient.

The same idea can be applied to patient flow. If patients arrive at an outpatient clinic at a steady rate that matches the clinic's ability to serve them, they can be seen in an efficient and consistent manner with little waiting. On the other hand, if they arrive in large surges, they are forced to wait, or the staff has to work harder or "cut corners" to process a large group of patients faster than usual, thereby compromising quality. This is why matching capacity to demand ("level loading") has such an impact on patient wait time and quality of care.

The process of consistently flowing patients is fundamental for allowing other aspects of a lean healthcare system to work. Figure 3.9 demonstrates that large surges of patients that unpredictably and unevenly enter the system can compromise the staff's ability to adhere to their care standards. However, level loading makes both minimal wait times and high quality possible.

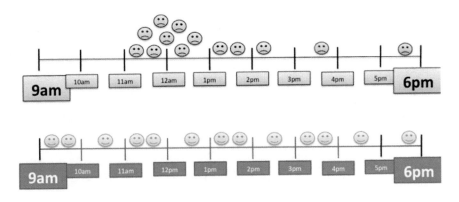

Figure 3.9: Patient flow before (top) and after (bottom) leveling

In addition to decreasing patient wait times (and the potential quality issues caused by hurried staff in response to unlevel patient demand), level loading patient flow can help dramatically reduce costs. Remember the water experiment? What were you doing the second time while waiting to take your next gulp? In all likelihood, you were doing nothing. This wasn't your fault, as there was nothing you could do but wait until the proper time to act. In healthcare settings, if you are paid by the hour, it's expensive to sit idle. This dynamic is played out each day when staff members wait for the rush of patients and then wait once the patient flow ceases. This imbalance has to be addressed to implement an advanced lean system.

Many critics believe that healthcare is unpredictable and not highly scheduled like manufacturing, so level loading is impossible. It is true that healthcare is subject to patient variability. For example, trauma patients are not scheduled in the emergency department; a spine surgery can take three hours longer than expected, thus disrupting the flow of patients into that operating room. In these instances, staff will need to be moved flexibly to areas of patient need to match capacity to demand. The variability necessitates a function like that of an air traffic controller, who makes adjustments for unforeseen variations in flight plans (Figure 3.10).

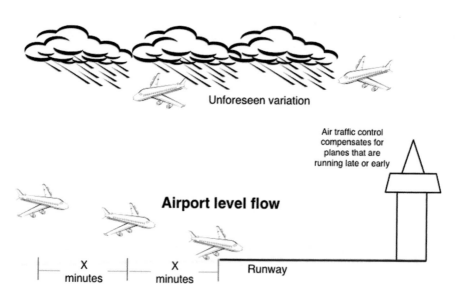

Figure 3.10: Air traffic control makes real-time adjustments where flow is not level

In practice, we find that most areas use a combination of leveling demand and flexible staffing to level capacity to demand. Patient flow can be leveled to a great degree in healthcare. If we standardize, level all that we can, and implement an "air traffic control" function to address unforeseen patient variability, capacity can be much more evenly matched to demand.

Building Quality into the System: Zero Defects Is the Only Acceptable Goal

Most people would agree that the only acceptable quality goal in healthcare is zero defects. Examples of defects include central-line infections, pressure ulcers, medication errors, reoperations, and readmissions. Although the "zero-defect" concept is ideal in theory, in practice, healthcare organizations serve up some of the worst quality results of any industry. Most healthcare quality metrics are measured in issues per hundred or thousand patients (e.g., three catheter infections per thousand catheter days), while most other industries have quality metrics measured in defects per million (e.g., three televisions per million have defective parts).

The current approach in healthcare is to try harder at improving quality by implementing protocols, training, audits, statistical analysis, impassioned emails, and endless meetings (an approach characterized by the joke, "The beatings will persist until morale improves"). A fresh approach is needed. Instead of aiming to make things slightly better, the focus should be on building processes that eliminate the possibility of errors in the first place. This zero-defect approach lies in stark contrast to the healthcare approach of merely trying to reduce quality occurrences.

To get started, we must first understand the conditions that cause quality defects. The first condition is human imperfection; errors will always be produced, even by the best people. The key is to accept this condition and implement a mindset and a set of strategies (e.g., error-proofing) to ensure that human error can never result in a patient-related quality issue. After a quality issue occurs, it is common for management to retrain staff on the "correct procedure." While this might help for a while, it can never completely prevent the issue from happening again, because human error is bound to occur sooner or later. Sadly, when the issue resurfaces, the competency of the staff is usually called into question instead of understanding that human error cannot be avoided. Implementing fixes with this "try harder" approach misses the point of accounting for human error when we want to solve quality issues.

Consider the everyday process of filling a non-diesel car with gasoline. Have you noticed that the diesel pump has a spout with a larger diameter than the gasoline spout? The size difference keeps you from making the mistake of filling your car with diesel. This is a good example of an error-proof process that will not allow human error to lead to a bad outcome. (Incidentally, you *can* put the smaller gasoline spout into a diesel tank, which has led to thousands of well-meaning people making a costly mistake.) Once we accept that human error is the cause of many quality issues, we must improve quality by implementing error-proofing mechanisms that do not allow human error to occur rather than demanding that people "try harder."

The second condition that leads to errors is that the healthcare system is set up such that "quality work" is an extra task. It needs to be built into the system. Take the example of the diesel spout; its diameter will not allow it to be placed in a non-diesel fuel tank. There is no extra step to use this spout, but it ensures that diesel is never put where it does not belong. If quality measures are not fully integrated into standardized work, adding steps to any process will not only be costly, but the organization will risk shortcuts around the new processes when the system is under stress.

The issue of healthcare workers washing their hands before and after contacting patients exemplifies this issue. Most workers know how important hand hygiene is, yet many report that they don't have enough time or access to hand washing stations. In this case, hand washing is an extra step that is commonly cut for the sake of efficiency. What if hand washing was integrated into the work (like the diesel spout) so that it was not an extra step?

Overview of the Lean Operating System: A System for Continuous Improvement

The following continuous improvement system lies at the heart of lean:

- Establish operational stability. Organize work areas with efficient layouts to ensure that staff, supplies, and equipment are available when needed.

- Level patient flow so that an area's resources can be efficiently used and their work standards can be maintained.
- Deliver just-in-time service so that staff and patients do not wait for what they need and there is neither lack nor excess of supplies, staff, or equipment.
- Ensure quality first so that no quality errors are passed on to the patient and the work environment is safe for the staff and clinicians.
- Where the system cannot meet these standards, continuously improve using the PDCA scientific method.

The basic "lean house" is a graphical representation of this operating system (Figure 3.11). Its pillars of quality first and just-in-time delivery are supported on a foundation of level patient flow and operational stability. This house will be "built" with more detail in chapter 4.

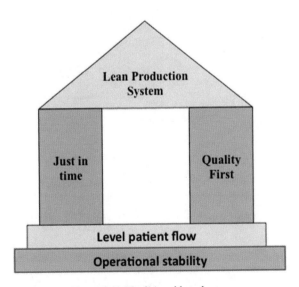

Figure 3.11: Traditional lean house

Lean has another important requirement, which is to continuously improve the system by engaging and developing the people doing the work. This is achieved by making abnormalities in processes visible, giving the team the proper time and coaching to improve their processes, addressing the root of problems, and eliminating waste so that the abnormalities don't recur. This approach requires leaders to take on the role of mentors and be tenacious about continuously improving processes with their teams. The healthcare environment has not been set up to work this way, so it is unreasonable to think that implementing a lean operating system will be possible without drastic changes.

Those changes are possible, and the next chapters explain how successful healthcare organizations have done it—and how you can too.

CHAPTER 4

The Lean Operating System: A Five-Level House

Lean is more than a set of tools or methods. In healthcare, it is a system of care delivery that focuses on creating value for the patient. As introduced in chapter two, this is accomplished by optimizing patient flow so that patients receive the highest quality care with no waiting and at a cost that is not prohibitive. Such optimization occurs *reliably* and *consistently* in a lean operating system.

Figure 4.1 depicts this system as a house, which is similar to the original Toyota Production System house (Figure 3.11). The house is a proxy for any healthcare enterprise: an inpatient hospital, an outpatient clinic, a private office, a subacute facility, or an outpatient surgery center.

The roof of the house represents the organization's true north: the organization's mission or *why* it is in business. In our model, it is to provide extraordinary patient care. Companies reach true north by attaining key performance indicators (KPIs) for quality and safety, timeliness, and a healing environment that confers maximal empathy to patients, all with the fewest possible resources (lowest cost). These true north metrics are designed so that individuals and teams have the tools to judge their own performance.

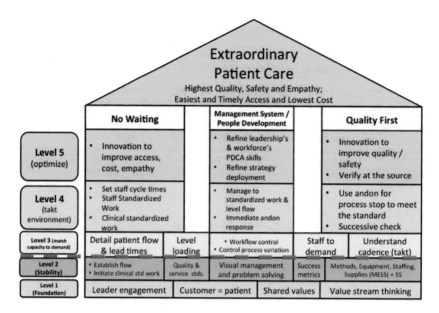

Figure 4.1: Advanced lean operating system

The three pillars and foundation show *how* true north is attained. This system supports the true north roof and is the framework for continuous improvement (PDCA cycles) using a set of tools, principles, and a people-development management system. This system aligns the organization around where it is, where it is going, and what it will take to get there.

The Quality first (or *Jidoka*) pillar, is the most important requirement of the system. The benchmark for quality in this system is perfection; anything less is unacceptable. The second pillar, No waiting (also termed "just in time"), represents the flow or efficiency of this system—how we ensure that healthcare workers and thus patients are not delayed in performing their duties or receiving care, respectively. The third pillar, daily management/people development, is not usually noted in traditional depictions of a lean system. The principles in this pillar are critical in creating lean engagement and alignment, developing capable problem solvers and leaders, and sustaining improvement gains. The house is "built" on five levels, each one representing a core lean principle; foundation, stability, match capacity to demand, takt environment, optimize. The lean principles depicted by the levels together comprise the lean operating system.

It is important to note that our depiction of a lean operating system is not meant to explain in detail the tools used for continuous improvement to achieve true north. Rather, the rectangular "boxes" within each level can be viewed as "drawers"—pull out any drawer to find the relevant tools and methodologies that can be used for continuous improvement at that level (e.g., A3 problem solving and 5S for organizing the workplace). The core principles and related tools are *introduced* at the various levels, but this does not mean that they are only used during work at that particular level. For example, understanding the eight types of waste occurs at level one, and waste elimination starts at level two, but expunging waste of all types continues throughout all the levels and in perpetuity.

Figure 4.2 emphasizes that working only on the basics (the blue rectangles), such as engagement and operational stability, will not be enough to transform healthcare from hockey to ballet. The entire operating system needs to change in a thoughtful, deliberate, and progressive manner.

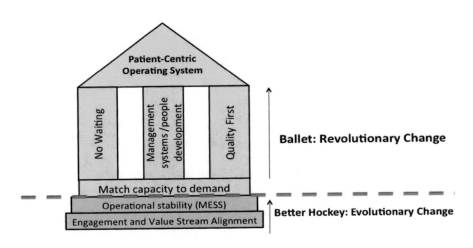

Figure 4.2: From hockey to ballet

The change represented by this figure can be broken into the following step-by-step approach, using the advanced lean operating system (Figure 4.3).

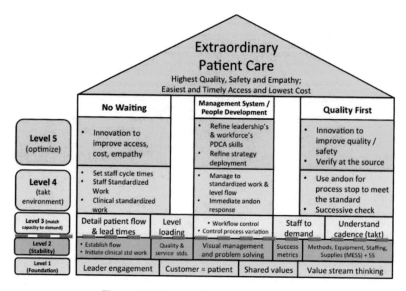

Figure 4.3: Advanced lean operating system

Level 1: Start by building a solid foundation and alignment

This step includes engaging and educating the staff, management, and clinicians in the journey. Most importantly, engage the senior executive team and physicians. From the outset, the team members must understand that the patient is the ultimate customer. They must understand that the key to everyone's long-term success is to share common values for a future state that produces the easiest access at the lowest cost and with the highest quality and empathy—as defined by the patient. To do this requires areas to be realigned by how *patients* flow through the healthcare system (using the value stream lens) instead of a traditional alignment around the clinicians' flow. Team members must agree to lower their guard enough to give this new approach a real chance to succeed. The only goal at this level is people development regarding education and alignment on a patient-centered system. (Level 1 is discussed in detail in chapter 5.)

Level 2: Create stability

Work areas need to be capable of reliable work before they are ready to move on to more advanced lean mechanisms. Gains garnered at this level are akin to playing better hockey. Readily available supplies, scheduling, equipment, staffing, work sequence, and workplace organization are examples of critical work elements. This concept is sometimes referred to as "methods, equipment, staffing and supplies" or MESS. This is where efforts to create flow within the operational areas are initiated and where managers learn how to be "lean leaders" by working with their teams to fix problems, using iterative PDCA cycles that hamper their everyday work. Along with implementing rudimentary process flows and workplace stability, this level is where much of the staff engagement and organizational lean learning occurs, because quality begins to increase while costs and wait times begin to decrease. Without implementing levels 1 and 2, progression to a more advanced lean state (ballet) is not possible. (Level 2 is discussed in detail in chapter 6.) This transformation objective is where most lean transformations in healthcare end.

Level 3: Match capacity to demand

This is where ballet begins, because tempo and scripting for patient flow need to be achieved. This defines the beginning of an advanced lean system. (The transition from hockey to ballet is denoted in figure 4.3 with a red dotted line between levels 2 and 3.) Once a clinical area's patient flow and lead times have been mapped (i.e., the value stream or clearly defined set of processes involved in meeting a patient's need), and the patient volume is understood, one can begin to match capacity to demand (level load) and calculate the cadence of patient demand (takt time). Important business structures need to be altered at this phase, including the implementation of a workflow control function at the workplace level, as well as long-term capacity and demand planning at the enterprise level. (The move from level 2 to level 3 is discussed in detail in chapter 7.)

Level 4: Implement a Takt Work Environment

Few healthcare institutions have achieved this step. At this level, the key work elements of the clinicians and staff are standardized, and management's job is to keep the team on cadence (takt) by real-time countermeasures for problems that stop patient flow. A process stop or "stop the line" mechanism is implemented so that procedure quality can be ensured along with consistent patient flow. At level 4, the volume of flagged abnormalities (issues that stop consistent patient flow) greatly increases, which requires a higher rate of problem solving on the part of management, staff, and clinicians than in previous levels. This phase lasts as long as it takes to become proficient at reliably hitting the required cadence of patient flow without defects in quality or patient experience. Substantial increases in quality and patient access, as well as decreases in costs and patient waiting times, are achieved at this level and continue through level 5. (Level 4 is discussed in detail in chapter 8.)

Level 5: Endlessly optimize standards

It is rare for any organization, healthcare or otherwise, to get to this point, which is the mark of an extremely mature lean system. This step is the crowning achievement of the Toyota Production System, which formed the basis for much of lean systems improvement thinking. Once a takt-driven environment (level 4) has been achieved, management works to reset (i.e., improve) the standards, resulting in standards that can no longer be achieved under the prior conditions. An example would be moving from a ninety-minute patient-recovery cadence in an OR recovery area to a new standard of eighty minutes. This new standard drives further improvement as the area staff work to become proficient at it. Once the new standard is achieved, the team continues to improve the standard and repeat in perpetuity. Level 5 is not a final step but an end state of continuous improvement. (Level 5 is discussed in detail in chapter 9.)

The Red Dotted Line between Levels 2 and 3

The red dotted line in our lean house graphic (Figure 4.3) depicts the critical transition between hockey and ballet. We added this line to emphasize that ballet begins above the line when patient flow and cadence begin to be achieved. This transition point also marks the biggest mental shift that needs to be overcome in traditional healthcare operations. Many management positions, which largely function as process expediters and "firefighters" (e.g., resource nurses) need to be retooled into workflow control and team lead entities (discussed in Chapter 8).

The Three Pillars: No Waiting, Daily Management System and People Development, Quality First

You may have noticed that the No Waiting and Quality First pillars of the lean healthcare house do not appear to extend all the way to the bottom in Figure 4.3. Three levels of foundation appear before they begin. However, this is not the case with the Daily Management System/People Development pillar. In figure 4.4, the thick lines depict where daily management or people development is occurring at each level. Level 1 dictates that at the start of a lean transformation, all resources should be dedicated to developing an organization's work force by creating alignment and shared values that place the patient at the center.

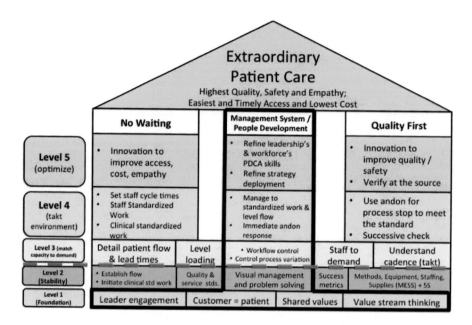

Figure 4.4: Advanced lean operating system – Management and People development

Do we have to wait for level 4 before working on No Waiting and Quality First? Things such as quality standards, establishing flow and stabilizing methods, staffing, equipment, and supplies have been implemented in level 2, so shouldn't the pillars start there?

The answer is not as simple as with the middle pillar. An organization may attain gains in reduced waiting and improved quality in early lean work, but they tend to occur sporadically and only very locally. At levels 2 and 3, the organization will lack the proper mechanisms to *ensure* that No Waiting and Quality First can be maintained, sustainably and system-wide. Without workload leveling (level 3), standardized work for staff (level 4), and process stop with management response (level 4), there may be pockets of No Waiting and Quality First, but they cannot reliably exist system-wide.

Three Critical Concepts Required for an Advanced Lean System (Levels 3 through 5)

Andon and Problem Solving

Using an *andon* to stop a process because of an abnormality can be confusing. An andon is a light, sound, colored flag, etc. that signals an abnormality. It is often used early in lean transformations (e.g., at Level 2) to record a problem with patient flow. These data are used to determine which improvements are needed. However, when an abnormality occurs in level 2 and an andon is signaled, patient flow typically does not stop, except when staff or patient safety is jeopardized. Instead the problem is noted, a quick countermeasure is implemented, and the patient continues on his or her journey.

By contrast, a mature lean system at level 4 has the supporting processes and management mindset to effectively use a "process stop" with an andon response. This means that patient flow completely stops—akin to shutting down an entire factory or operating room—this stoppage ensures a rapid management response such that a quick countermeasure is implemented and the patient's journey proceeds as described above. Management is then tasked with understanding the root cause so that the issue can be solved. Then a quick countermeasure is implemented and the patient's journey proceeds as described above. The key difference between these Level 2 and Level 4 scenarios is a mindset change from solely implementing quick countermeasures to root cause problem solving. The organization must have mature problem-solving processes in place to attack the problem (the quality defect) identified by the process stop, with the thought of preventing it from happening again.

Let's use hand hygiene to illustrate this concept. Excellent data support the contention that proper hand hygiene minimizes patient and staff infections (a topic receiving national attention at the time of this writing). Many organizations start a campaign to get their workers to wash their hands; they create the burning platform and align around the cause (level 1), create standards, train to those standards, and manage to those standards while introducing daily audits (level 2). Despite these actions, many practitioners still don't wash their hands 100 percent of the time. There is no system to prevent them from touching patients if they don't wash unless they are caught by an auditor (andon) or a concerned colleague. This level 2 system is not reliable, it costs money (in auditor time), and is difficult to scale. The problem is not solved at its root.

At a lean level 4, root cause problem solving for noncompliance would be a system where, for example, the clinician could not enter a patient's room due to a physical barrier linked to hand washing. This is a true process stop, because the practitioner cannot proceed with patient care without washing.

The authors acknowledge that process stop can occur earlier than level four, such as in level 2. For example, a patient with heart disease may be noted, on the morning of surgery, to have an incomplete work-up for the planned procedure. This patient cannot undergo anesthesia and surgery, so the process (patient flow) is stopped. However, it is still incumbent upon the system to move from level 2 immediate countermeasure problem solving (e.g., have a cardiologist see the patient and then the surgery is performed later that same day) to a level 4 system so that the problem is solved at its root and never happens again (e.g., a pre-anesthesia clinic screens all patients of a certain risk classification so that incomplete work-ups never occur).

Time

One of the most powerful tools in the lean operating system is time. Understanding how long a given process takes, and then ensuring that staff and clinicians have the proper time available to do the task, is fundamental to a high-functioning, lean operating system. This system, as depicted by the house in Figure 4.3, identifies time in the forms of takt time (level 3), patient lead times (level 3) and staff cycle times (level 4).

At first blush, specifying times for how long processes should take may seem far too mechanistic for a healthcare setting. The thought of clinicians working like robots to a metronome's pace paints a disturbing mental picture. In practice, timed work efforts offer the staff and clinicians the opposite. For example, when a time-based nursing standard is set for inpatient room rounding, it gives the nurse a way to ask for help when she is not allowed the proper time to do the job at hand. It is important that management and the nursing staff, together, set the standardized time for the rounding. Thus, there is agreement that a high quality workflow (in this case, room rounds) will take a given time, which forces the team to solve the issues that impede the staff from having the proper time to do their jobs.

Another attribute of time is abnormality detection. Asking "Did the expected steps get completed in the allotted time?" is among the easiest and most reliable ways to detect if the system is performing as expected. When a process cannot meet its standardized time, it signals that continuous improvement should be applied so that the next time the process is performed, it can meet the standard.

Leadership

Although the terms executives, senior management, and area management—and their respective roles—may vary from organization to organization, we define them, as they pertain to a stable lean organization, as follows.

- **Area management: Staff with direct operations (line) management responsibility.**
  Their job is to set the standards, with their staff, for their area of responsibility and enable the staff to attain those standards. Area managers spend the majority of their day in the workplace where value is created for patients (the gemba), supporting frontline workers.

- **Senior management: Organizational leaders who do not have direct line management responsibility.**
  Their job is to help area managers solve the issues causing deviations from standards (that is, to support a stable operating system). Senior managers spend less time in the gemba than area managers, but they still practice going to the gemba to see the issues and the progress being made against them, on a daily basis.

- **Executives: Highest organizational leaders who occupy the "C-suite" (the CEO, COO, CFO, etc.).**
  Ninety percent of executives' time is focused on strategic initiatives. During the other 10 percent, they support a stable operating system, as do senior management, by going to the gemba on a daily basis, seeing the issues, and supporting improvement efforts.

Leadership and staff both undergo transformation during a lean implementation. The leadership triangle captures the progressive movement from a management-by-objectives (MBO) mentality (with the CEO at top of the triangle and all others below) to a servant leadership mentality (with the CEO and management at bottom, serving the frontline workers, who are at the top). Figure 4.5 illustrates this principle.

Leadership Triangle	Executive Objectives	Senior Manager Objectives	Area Manager Objectives	Staff & Clinician Objectives
Level 5	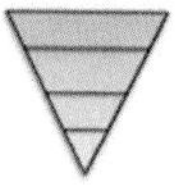 • Mature demand and capacity planning • Coach in gemba enterprise-wide	• Continuous improvement via cycle time reduction • Daily continuous improvement • Implement error proofing	• Manage cycle time reduction • Daily improvement with staff against issues that impede flow • Implement error proofing	• Adhere to standardized work • Andon when standardized work cannot be met • Root-cause solve issues that impede flow
Level 4	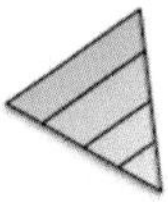 • Enterprise-wide goal, deployment mature • Continue gemba rounds (coach in VS and help staff fix problems)	Implement: • Immediate andon response • Standardized work • Efficiency graphs assessment	• Implement team lead • Immediate andon response • Verify standardized work adherence • Efficiency graphs to manage pt. flow	• Adhere to standardized work • Andon when standardized work cannot be met • Root-cause solve issues that impede flow

Level 3	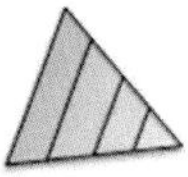 • Implement VS demand and capacity planning
	• Understand VS, takt
	• Continue gemba rounds
		• Calculate takt
		• Implement production control
		  • Capacity & demand planning
		  • Level scheduling
		  • Air traffic control
			• Staff to leveled schedule (day before)
			• Adjust staffing to actual demand (day of)
				• Staff begins to feel more consistent workload

Level 2	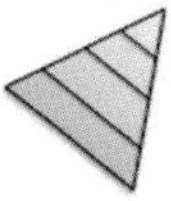 • Begin managing by VS • Help solve issues in the gemba	• Patient flow owned by one entity (senior mgr.) • Senior mgr.'s primary responsibility is to fix all issues that impede patient flow • Coach in the gemba	• Coach in the gemba • Maintain MESS • Shift from managing people to managing processes • Respond to staff issues	• Staff feels mgmt.'s presence • Support through MESS improvements • Begin to surface issues with daily work
Level 1	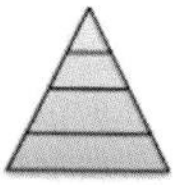 • Study trips & lean education • Go see issues • Customer (value stream) alignment	• No value stream (patient flow) alignment • Groups managed in silos by lines of authority	• Daily work largely driven by MBO requirements • Respond to area emergencies (triage)	• Staff feels minimal support from mgmt. • Limited ability to improve area

VS = value stream; MBO = managing by objectives
MESS = methods, equipment, staffing, supplies
Figure 4.5: Lean leadership levels (*See page 240 for expanded view of figure 4.5)

Leaders develop themselves and their workers by asking these questions: "What problem are we trying to solve?" "What is the current state of the process leading to this problem?" "What is your desired future state?" "How can the organization best help you and your colleagues reach this state?"

Leaders are required to be good listeners and humble students so that they can deeply understand the issue, coach, and develop the workers on root cause problem solving. Developing an army of problem solvers allows waste and unnecessary variation of processes to be removed in order to reach the organization's true north and related KPIs (quality, safety, access, empathy, cost). This transition will be explained in chapter 5.

We would like share a story told by economic expert Ernesto Sirolli.[11] Without referring explicitly to "lean leadership techniques," he tells a story, in plain terms, of what it means to be a lean leader: Go to the gemba, listen more than you talk, ask more then you tell, support the folks who are content experts, work with the local staff to solve problems, and empower people based on their mission-centric passion.

Sirolli recounted the years 1971–1977 during which he worked for an Italian nongovernmental organization in Africa. He is a noted authority in the field of sustainable economic development and the founder of the Sirolli Institute, an international nonprofit organization that helps local communities help themselves.

Sirolli began his talk by saying, "Every single project we set up in Africa failed. I was distraught. I thought that we Italians were good people and we were doing good work in Africa. Instead, everything we touched, we killed." His first project in Africa was teaching people in Zambia how to grow tomatoes, zucchini, and other Italian favorites. He shares, "Instead of asking them why they were not growing anything, we simply said, 'Thank God we're here.'" With little help from the Zambians, his team planted vegetables in the lush, fertile Zambian soil—there could not be a better environment for agriculture. As predicted, the crops grew remarkably well, but as harvesting time approached, the Italians watched in horror as two hundred hippos stormed out of a nearby river and ate everything in sight. All of a sudden, Sirolli understood why the locals hadn't been interested in growing food.

Sirolli said that aid from Western countries tends to come in two forms: paternalistic (I treat you like my son) and patronizing (I treat you like my servant). After decades working in international aid, he had seen that neither worked. He championed a type of aid that he called enterprise facilitation.

"The first principle of aid is respect," he said. "If people do not wish to be helped, leave them alone. You become a servant of the local passion, of local people who have a dream to become a better person. What you do is you shut up, you never arrive in a community with any ideas, and you sit with the local people, not in offices. Become friends. Find out what that person wants to do. You have to create a new profession—be the family doctor of enterprise who sits with you in your house at the kitchen table and helps you find the resources to transform your passion into a way to make a living. It is important to cultivate each person's passion, for personal growth, give them support for their ideas, and help them develop the knowledge necessary for personal therefore organizational growth. Don't arrive and tell them what to do."

Sirolli has gone on to help people in many ways. The Italian government once asked him about his success, "How did you do that?" He said, "I shut up and listen to the people. You have to learn to get people to come and talk to you. You have to be fantastic at helping them, and then they will come in droves. Offer them dedicated and impassioned service. You can change the culture of the community just by capturing the passion, energy, and imagination of your own people."

Advanced Lean Operating System and KPIs (True North Metrics)

Patient Experience

Gains in the patient experience can be broken down in terms of quality, access, cost, and empathy. Creating extraordinary patient care (the true north of the house) is analogous to consistently delivering extraordinary patient experience. As an organization ascends the levels of the house, it is able to *reliably* deliver a better patient experience. Figure 4.6 outlines this progression.

	Consistent Patient Experience	Easiest Access	Highest Quality	Lowest Cost	Highest Empathy
Level 5	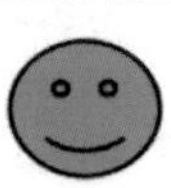	• Shortest wait times and fastest service through continuous improvement lead time improvement	• Highest quality stemming from increasing amount of error proofing (i.e., source inspection)	• Lowest overall system cost through continuous cycle time improvement (~30%) • Significant opportunity to pass savings onto customer	• Highest level of compassion through continuous improvement of standard (courtesy, respect, listening, responsiveness, special touches)
Level 4	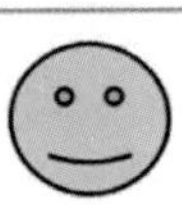	• Additional decrease in wait times due to following standardized work and meeting takt	• Significant increase in quality from building quality into staff standardized work: • Consistent processes • Line stop • Self-inspection	• Continue to significantly reduce overall system cost (~30%) • Growing opportunity to pass savings to customer	• Build empathy into staff standard work resulting in higher levels of : • Courtesy • Respect • Listening • Responsiveness
Level 3	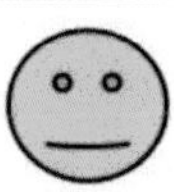	• Significant decrease in wait times due to: • Capacity and demand planning • Level scheduling • Air traffic control	• Increased quality via: • Consistent cadence, allowing time for staff to focus on patient	• Begin to significantly reduce overall system cost (~10%) • Opportunity to pass savings to customer	• Increased opportunity for empathy and special touches via a consistent cadence, allowing time for staff to focus on patient
Level 2	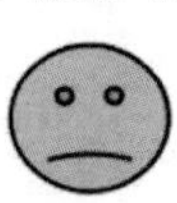	• Slightly decreased wait times due to improved: • Staffing • Scheduling • Fewer barriers via VS alignment • Language • Transportation	• Quality slightly increased via: • Quality gates • Audits • Work standards	• Reduce overall system cost slightly (~5%)	• Slightly increased opportunity for compassion and special touches via: • DMS • Problem solving • Visual management
Level 1	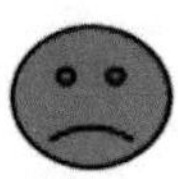	• System inconsistency results in long wait times • Scheduled appts. • Waiting room • Transportation difficulties • Language barriers	• System inconsistency results in high occurrence of : • HAI's • Medical errors • Incorrect information • Poor handoffs • Many work-arounds	• System inconsistency results in high cost • Service is too expensive	• System inconsistency results in lack of: • Courtesy, respect, listening, responsiveness • No time for special touches

VS = Value Stream; DMS = Daily Management System

Figure 4.6: Patient experience levels (*See page 241 for expanded view of figure 4.6)

Quality and Safety Improvements

Positive effects of ascending the levels of the house can be seen in quality and safety. The operational stability that characterizes level 2 starts positively transforming quality and safety by making the organization capable of catching quality and safety problems before they are discovered by the patient, albeit at the last step of the process. In level 3, matching capacity to demand improves quality and safety by allowing the staff to work at a reasonable and consistent pace rather than hurrying during spikes in patient demand. In a level 4 takt environment, the staff and clinicians on the unit can consistently check themselves as they do their work and practice process stop where the standard cannot be met. Finally, level 5 supplies the infrastructure necessary to redesign the processes so that quality and safety errors cannot occur. Figure 4.7 outlines this progression.

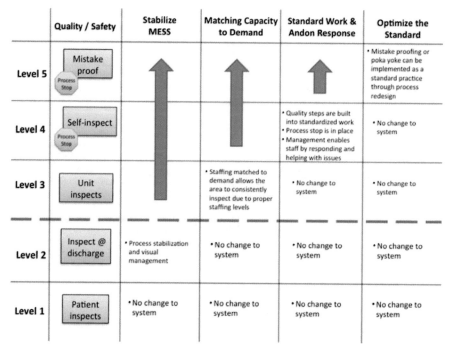

	Quality / Safety	Stabilize MESS	Matching Capacity to Demand	Standard Work & Andon Response	Optimize the Standard
Level 5	Mistake proof (Process Stop)				• Mistake proofing or poka yoke can be implemented as a standard practice through process redesign
Level 4	Self-inspect (Process Stop)			• Quality steps are built into standardized work • Process stop is in place • Management enables staff by responding and helping with issues	• No change to system
Level 3	Unit inspects		• Staffing matched to demand allows the area to consistently inspect due to proper staffing levels	• No change to system	• No change to system
Level 2	Inspect @ discharge	• Process stabilization and visual management	• No change to system	• No change to system	• No change to system
Level 1	Patient inspects	• No change to system	• No change to system	• No change to system	• No change to system

Figure 4.7: Quality and safety levels (*See page 242 for expanded view of figure 4.7)

Cost Benefits

Cost benefits come in a variety of ways in both clinical and nonclinical departments: cost reduction (hard dollars that can be realized one time or recurring), cost avoidance (potential dollars), and revenue increases (potential or hard dollars). For example, hard dollars would result from worker productivity improvements, decrease in inventory, and decrease in the use of premium labor and travelers. Cost avoidance can result from decreasing space needs, doing more in the same or less space, retaining talented workers, and fewer lawsuits due to better clinical quality. Revenue increases can result from a more efficient revenue cycle and increased clinical capacity or backfill opportunities if the organization has a strategic plan to grow its business.

Let's examine cost reduction with respect to the levels of the house (Figure 4.8).

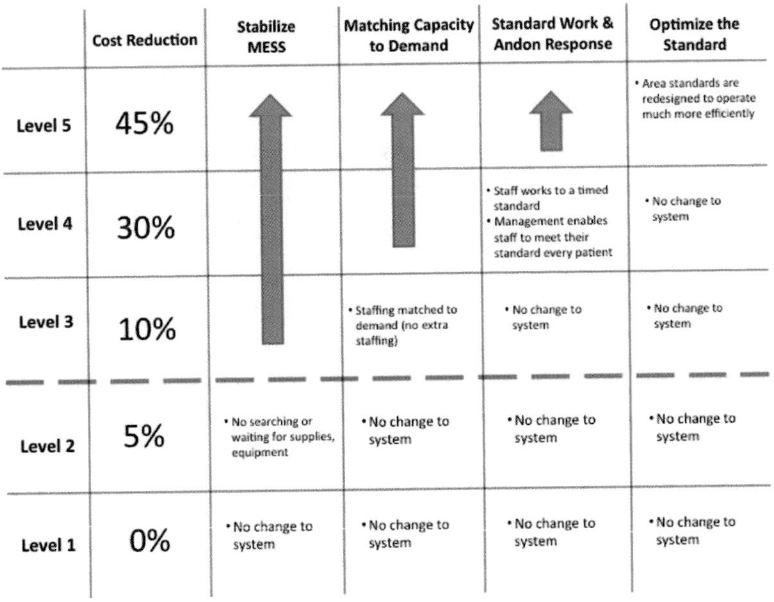

	Cost Reduction	Stabilize MESS	Matching Capacity to Demand	Standard Work & Andon Response	Optimize the Standard
Level 5	45%				• Area standards are redesigned to operate much more efficiently
Level 4	30%			• Staff works to a timed standard • Management enables staff to meet their standard every patient	• No change to system
Level 3	10%		• Staffing matched to demand (no extra staffing)	• No change to system	• No change to system
Level 2	5%	• No searching or waiting for supplies, equipment	• No change to system	• No change to system	• No change to system
Level 1	0%	• No change to system	• No change to system	• No change to system	• No change to system

Figure 4.8: Cost reduction levels (*See page 243 for expanded view of figure 4.8)

The ability to garner greater cost reductions occurs as an organization "ascends" in the lean house. Level 2 work allows for some cost reduction in the form of reduced searching and waiting for supplies and equipment as well as a one time savings in the form of inventory reduction. Supply chain replenishment systems, such as kanban, are implemented at level 2, and these systems allow an organization to reduce stock outs, par levels, and obsolescence costs. They also allow for basic improvements in patient flow and reduced waiting times, thus increasing capacity to care for more patients. Although these cost reduction improvements aren't trivial, they offer relatively small gains compared to what can be accomplished at levels 3, 4, and 5 (ballet). Level 3's larger cost reduction potential lies in the ability to match capacity to demand, which avoids some overstaffing costs even though the staff isn't yet working at their optimal output. In level 4, the staff and clinicians are working to a particular cadence (a takt environment), which implies two things: staffing matches patient flow, and staff and clinicians complete their work in a standardized amount of time. Driving more waste out of the system, coupled with staff being able to perform their tasks within the allotted time (level 4) allows the organization to care for more patients.

When the authors started level 4 work in one area of our organization, we found that, on average, only 29 percent of the expected work output was reliably accomplished. Said another way, as the area became proficient at achieving takt time goals, they reduced the total costs (including labor) by a whopping 245 percent! Although level 3 and 4 offer substantial cost reduction opportunities, level 5 work centers on redesigning the work so that even more waste can be removed. These revolutionary changes can drastically reduce or eliminate the work required to do the same job, and the continuous improvement approach at level 5 will yield cost reductions in perpetuity.

Overview

Now that the changes in leadership, cost, quality, safety, and patient experience have been outlined, we can combine them. Figure 4.9 depicts the changes in each category as an organization ascends through the levels of the house.

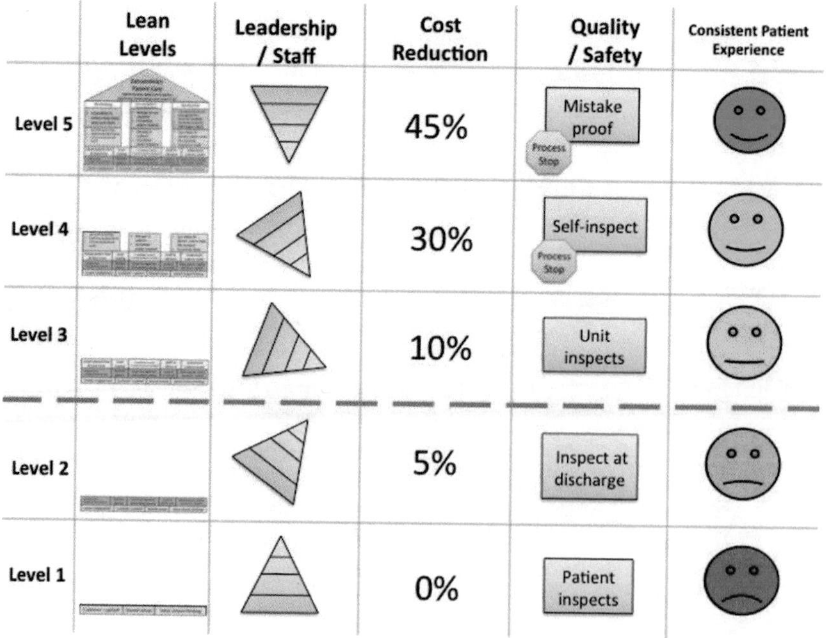

Figure 4.9: Advanced lean transformation overview
(*See page 244 for expanded view of figure 4.9)

Figure 4.9 also can be used as a diagnostic tool for understanding at what level a given area is currently operating. For example, the staff and management of an area may be operating at level three with their daily management and methods, but if the executives who oversee that area are only managing at level two (see figure 4.5 on lean leadership levels) then the area's overall level of operation is level 2. It is important to note that getting an area to the "next level" will not occur until all parties (from executives to the front line staff and clinicians) are simultaneously working and managing at the same level. Therefore, it is the lowest level of operation of any part of an area that determines its overall level of performance.

Implementing the House Is a Nonlinear Affair

Although the levels of the advance lean operating system house might seem to imply a step-by-step, linear approach (complete level 1 and move to level 2, etc.), as depicted in figure 4.10a, in practice this could not be further from the truth. Lean transformations undergo a lot of seesawing between levels. This is natural and, in fact, required. As the organization's lean understanding grows and people gain more experience by working on higher levels, the organization recognizes things that should have been done at previous levels, causing a seesaw effect.

For example, let's say that an inpatient unit believes it is operating at level 4. When a nurse is discharging a patient, she realizes that transportation has not been set up, so she stops the process and signals the abnormality with an andon, such as an immediate page to a manager. Management responds immediately and helps to fix the problem. Although stopping the process and the immediate management response are level 4 activities, this situation points out a problem with having a stable and reliable transport method (which should have been addressed earlier in the area's level 2 stability work). This does not mean that the area is wrongly doing level 4 work before it has completed level 2; it just points out a deeper understanding of what each level is trying to accomplish. In this case, the team would "jump" back to level 2, conduct an improvement activity on creating a stable transport process, implement it, and return to the level 4 work it was doing before. This natural seesawing is depicted in figure 4.10b.

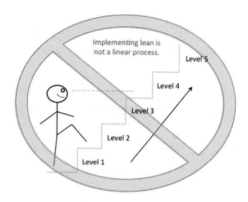

Figure 4.10a: Perceived step-by-step progression

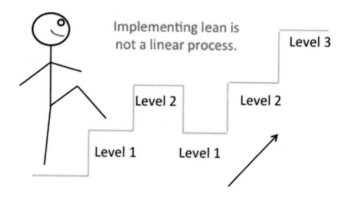

Figure 4.10b: Actual progression is a seesaw between levels

As you read this book, keep in mind the requirements for continuous improvement such as leadership, patient experience, staff experience, quality, and timeliness as well as the nonlinear nature of the actual implementation process. From this point forward, each chapter gives the maximum amount of detail so that you can formulate a plan for an advanced lean transformation in your organization.

CHAPTER 5

Level 1–Create the Foundation through Engagement and Shared Values

Extraordinary Patient Care					
Highest Quality, Safety and Empathy; Easiest and Timely Access and Lowest Cost					

	No Waiting		**Management System / People Development**	**Quality First**	
Level 5 (optimize)	• Innovation to improve access, cost, empathy		• Refine leadership's & workforce's PDCA skills • Refine strategy deployment	• Innovation to improve quality / safety • Verify at the source	
Level 4 (takt environment)	• Set staff cycle times • Staff Standardized Work • Clinical standardized work		• Manage to standardized work & level flow • Immediate andon response	• Use andon for process stop to meet the standard • Successive check	
Level 3 (match capacity to demand)	Detail patient flow & lead times	Level loading	• Workflow control • Control process variation	Staff to demand	Understand cadence (takt)
Level 2 (Stability)	• Establish flow • Initiate clinical std work	Quality & service stds.	Visual management and problem solving	Success metrics	Methods, Equipment, Staffing, Supplies (MESS) + 5S
Level 1 (Foundation)	Leader engagement	Customer = patient	Shared values	Value stream thinking	

In chapter 2, we emphasized that lean in healthcare is a system predicated on quality—nothing is more important for this industry. We discussed the relation of quality and value and emphasized that the patient is the customer in healthcare. In chapter 3, we reviewed key lean fundamentals including the importance of value stream thinking, and in chapter 4, we described the details of the five-level house.

We are now ready to build the house starting with the foundation. To fully describe level 1, we start by again emphasizing that the patient is the customer. We review the importance of thinking about the patients as they move "horizontally" through the value streams of the healthcare system (not in vertical silos). We focus heavily on shared values that allow us to define true north, which in turn allows us to create organizational alignment around shared needs and goals. With shared values, goals, and organizational alignment, the organization can truly engage its workforce, beginning with its leaders.

This chapter is the longest in the book and deservedly so. We found that without spending ample time building the foundation, the operating system (or rest of the house) will be unstable. It is critical to understand that the speed and depth of implementation depends on organizational alignment, particularly at the senior executive level. Without this alignment, the lean implementation will be slow, may fail to progress beyond level 2 (most commonly), or may completely fail and be abandoned. It is important to note that once an organization embarks on a lean journey, levels 1 and 2 tend to commence simultaneously. Education and alignment begin to occur, problems that are hindering value creation for the organization's patients are agreed upon, and the work of attaining basic stability or MESS commences.

The Patient Is Our Customer

In a healthcare organization, the customer is not the physician specialist, the nurse, or the referring provider—it is always the patient. From a philosophical standpoint, we never get significant pushback on this point. From a practical standpoint, however, agreement isn't so universal.

If you look at our systems of care, they are often designed around maximizing efficiency for the providers. In general, optimizing systems around providers doesn't result from selfish motives. Rather, optimization evolves based on a false notion that optimizing for a scarce resource (the providers) results in more efficient patient care. In reality, when optimization occurs around the scarce resource, the result is batching, and patients often end up waiting. As an example, many medical teams in a hospital enter orders only after all rounds have been completed. Batching orders in this way can be more efficient for senior members of the rounding team—they can get on to the next task more quickly. The issue is that batching orders results in patients waiting, delays in care, and potentially longer hospital stays.

To acknowledge that the patient is the customer means that value in a healthcare organization is defined only by the patient. When there is a choice between optimizing a process for patient flow or provider efficiency, the patient flow must take precedence. Provider efficiency is important, but it never trumps value for the customer.

Value Stream Thinking

Value Streams Focus an Organization on Optimizing Patient Flow

The ultimate goal of any lean business system is to exceed customer expectations. To accomplish this goal, lean organizations relentlessly work to improve the flow of value to their customers. It comes as no surprise that the ease with which patients move through the care continuum drives a large part of their satisfaction. Because patients are our customers in healthcare and they alone define value, if a healthcare organization hopes to be successful, it must focus on how patients flow through the system. This stands in contrast to the traditional focus of optimizing efficiency in isolated work areas (a procedure unit, the medical records department, a physician's office, etc.).

The "value stream approach" (outlined in chapters 2 and 3) needs to be applied to all areas of an organization to optimize quality and the patient experience and to discover the greatest areas of waste. As seen in the figure 5.1, the value stream approach centers on optimizing patient flow from start to finish regardless of the care that the patients receive. Each step of the journey should be planned and optimized through lean methodologies so that patients receive the best access, best quality, and highest empathy, all at the lowest cost.

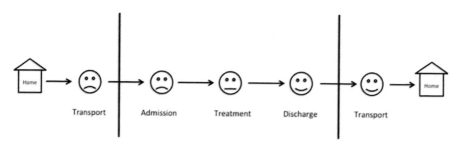

Figure 5.1: Value stream flow = patient flow

Traditional Thinking Is "Siloed Thinking"

Traditionally, clinicians and managers have worked on optimizing work processes in their own area, which leads to localized efficiency but does not create the patient-centered value stream flow required in a complex healthcare system.

To illustrate the problem of siloed thinking, let's consider a twenty-member symphonic orchestra. These professionals are highly trained and experienced musicians. Imagine them coming together on stage, their roles nicely scripted on their sheet music. However, instead of starting and stopping in a well-choreographed way, taking into consideration those who play before and after each other, they all start playing at random times. Each one plays the section beautifully, but together, it is nothing more than noise. They are using their talents to generate music at their own cadence but disregarding the effect on the other musicians.

This siloed approach does not work for an orchestra, and the same is true for clinicians working hard at their care delivery sub-processes (their sheet music or script). They have little regard to the upstream or downstream effects of their work, which could result in a suboptimal patient experience (bad music or simply noise).

Shared Values

True North and Creating Alignment

In every business, three entities must be satisfied simultaneously: the customer (the patient), the corporation, and the workers (the clinicians and staff).

The needs of each group are not equal, but the patient's needs are paramount—their requirements result in the organization's true north. That said, all three must see gains from engaging in a lean enterprise for the maximum effect to be realized. Like a three-legged stool (Figure 5.2), understanding that all three legs, not just one or two, are required is the first step in getting the lean enterprise to work properly.

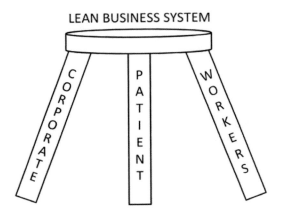

LEAN BUSINESS SYSTEM

Figure 5.2: Lean business system

Patient Needs (True North)

As stated earlier, a patient wants many things from the healthcare experience. We will focus on the items that transcend all patient strata; high-quality care, low cost, timely access, and high empathy. Together these elements define extraordinary patient care, and in a healthcare organization, there is no higher purpose. Care that is high in quality, high in empathy, timely, and low in cost is the true north of a healthcare organization. These needs are consistent across all patient types, because all patients want extraordinary care.

Though we depicted true north as the roof of a lean operating "house" in chapter 4, another way to represent true north, as well as the requirements for the three-legged stool, is shown in what we refer to as the birthday cake-type diagram. We build the cake by starting with true north (Figure 5.3):

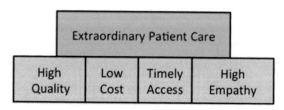

Figure 5.3: Lean goal "true north"

As described in chapter 4, extraordinary patient care is the organization's mission, and the metrics or KPIs in purple, if met, allow the organization to reach its true north.

Manager's, Clinician's, and Staff Needs

To be successful, people who work in a healthcare system need to feel that a lean transformation will benefit them as they strive to provide extraordinary patient care. Just as patients have needs, workers have fundamental needs: meaningful work, a reasonable workload, to feel supported by the management, a consistent "good" income, and a culture of respect in a safe work environment. These relationships stack as additional layers of the birthday cake diagram (Figure 5.4):

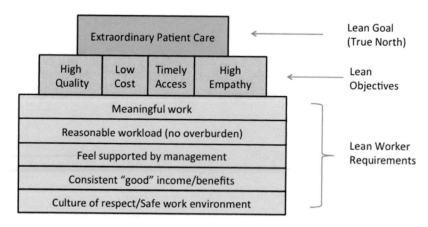

Figure 5.4: Patient and worker needs

It is important to pay special attention to getting clinicians, particularly physicians, to understand how a lean transformation will help them so that they embrace the process as soon as possible. This is not because clinicians are more important than other workers, but it is an acknowledgement that perhaps they are the most siloed. "Point improvements" (lean improvements that address discrete problems, often in a discrete area of the organization) can be effective in engaging workers of all types, including physicians. Aside from the workers making the improvement themselves, point improvements can help build teams and demonstrate how lean works. It is important to start by removing the waste that each stakeholder group sees as opportunities for improvement.

Typical candidates for point improvements are as follows:

1. Workplace organization
2. Supply readiness
3. Equipment readiness
4. Removal of unnecessary steps in defined processes
5. Visual management of processes and outcomes
6. Staffing plan stability and creating consistent shifts and breaks for staff

Engaging the Staff at All Levels

It is critical to use lean transformation to inspire passion in the organization's employees concerning their personal growth, because lean requires a tenacious, hands-on approach for everyone (especially senior operations and clinical management). Failing to get leaders to become active lean advocates is the cause of nearly all lean transformation failures.

If we reflect on Johnny's story in chapter 1, there were many points along the way that leadership could have intervened to help the flow of Johnny's discharge but did not. In fact, from the senior manager's point of view, the discharge looked "normal." He/she would have never given it another thought. This is why observing the work personally is so critical. When people are passionate about their personal growth, they become engaged in the processes. When passion is lacking, people disengage. Figures 5.5a–c depict the problem associated with disengaged senior management. The angle that the boulder (representing patient experience) needs to navigate represents the degree of leadership engagement.

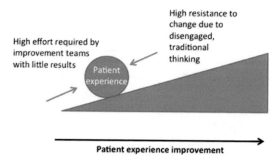

Figure 5.5a: High effort with small improvement

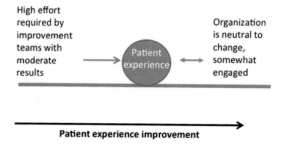

Figure 5.5b: High effort with moderate improvement

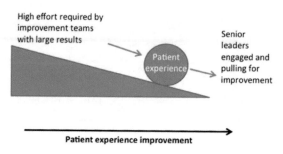

Figure 5.5c: High effort with high improvement

As these figures show, the degree of engagement at the senior levels determines how quickly the patient experience improves and how much improvement effort will be needed. This is why creating a vision that all levels agree to and feel invested in must be the first step.

Corporate Needs

Without a strong financial footing, no organization can achieve its goals. Profitability and affordability are fundamental concepts when discussing the finances of an organization. From our point of view, profitability and affordability are closely related, but optimizing for one or the other has different implications. Patients and third-party payers (employers, insurers, and the government) seek affordability, which exists within the greater context of the market. In the healthcare system in the United States, if a provider is not affordable, patients will be directed (or will direct themselves) to another system. Strictly speaking, being affordable doesn't equate with being profitable; a service can be provided at a loss that, if large enough, will risk the sustainability of the organization. For this reason, the corporation seeks profitability.

In healthcare, the predominant strategy for making profit has been based on growing market share (acting like a revenue center), because the industry has traditionally been able to set prices. As a consequence, the industry has not substantially focused on reliably and sustainably controlling costs (acting like an expense center). However, as the market becomes more competitive due to limitations placed on healthcare spending, affordable pricing will become increasingly important. If healthcare is forced to become more affordable, organizations will need to focus on waste reduction as a sustainable path for continued profitability.

In reality, generating more revenue (increasing patient volume) and decreasing cost (diminishing waste) are performed concurrently. Lean businesses, however, demonstrate that the only way to long-term, sustainable profitability is through cost reduction. In a lean business, the way to generate more revenue is to be more affordable than the competition without sacrificing quality and while still generating a profit. This paradigm shift is relevant for the healthcare industry as organizations, and hospitals in particular, move from viewing themselves as revenue centers to expense centers. Expense management through waste elimination, inextricably coupled with high quality and exceptional experience, forms the basis of lean improvement.

As the healthcare reform flourishes, it becomes increasing difficult for systems to pass on increasing costs to customers by demanding a price. Lean thinking aligns nicely with the notion that the market controls prices (value-based purchasing) and advocates that the best way to garner a profit is to reduce costs through continuous improvement. Two profit-gaining systems are depicted in Figure 5.6 below:

Profit = Price - Cost Lean thinking: The patient/payer (i.e. market) has control over the price, so the way to increase profit is to reduce costs.	**Price = Cost + Profit** Traditional thinking: The business has control over the price, so the business can increase profit by increasing prices.

Figure 5.6: Profit equation; Lean vs. Traditional view

The equation in the left box implies a cost-conscious attitude in the organization. The equation in the right box implies that whatever a service costs, it will be sold at a higher price. This selfish approach to business flies in the face of an organization's obligation to serve society.

As far back as Aristotle, philosophers have remarked that humans are fundamentally social animals. Lean organizations embrace this aspect of human nature and, on a corporate basis, acknowledge the responsibility to contribute positively to society. Doing so is a potent motivator for employees and is viewed favorably by customers. In healthcare, contributing to society is naturally performed by virtue of the value that the organization generates. Disease treatment and prevention, accident prevention, health education programs, charity care, community outreach and sponsorship, and patient advocacy initiatives are some of the ways that a healthcare system can and do contribute to society.

Incorporating the lean corporate requirement of profitability through cost reduction and its contributions to society as a whole, our lean business system can be viewed in the following way, with the lean corporate requirements completing the layers of the birthday cake diagram (Figure 5.7):

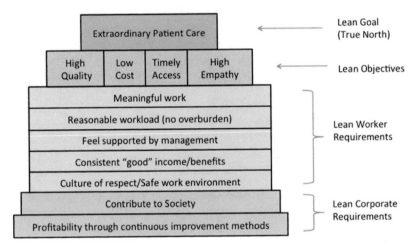

Figure 5.7: Shared values "Birthday cake"

Figure 5.7 outlines what prosperity (shared values) for all three entities (patient, workers, corporate) looks like in a lean enterprise. Most importantly, everyone in the organization needs to understand the true north alignment or value statement.

Leadership Requirements

The primary job of a lean leader is to support the frontline work so that the patient needs can be met with as little effort as possible. Leaders also have the responsibility of hiring and growing the next generation of leaders so that when the time comes, new leadership can take over seamlessly (succession planning). We use words like *help, mentor, coach, grow,* and *support frontline work* to describe the attributes of a lean leader. In a lean system, a leader's primary role is to serve as a helper or enabler, not an order giver.

Dive Deep into Defects

The basis of lean systems is to set standards so that defects (deviations from the standard) can be detected and improved. We find that setting up systems to reveal defects is relatively easy; responding to and root cause fixing the defect is hard.

To get started, we must redefine the leader's daily work. In a lean system, leaders are enablers (helpers). They remove the barriers that the frontline workers encounter as they work to their established standards. As defects pop up, it is the leader's job to solve these issues so that they don't impede the frontline staff's work cycles. Getting to the root of problems takes "diving deep into the weeds" and spending the time to ensure that issues are completely resolved before moving on. It is critical that leaders at all organizational levels understand that their primary responsibility is removing the barriers that impede care by understanding problems. Without this understanding, lean leaders cannot develop, and the staff cannot develop as problem solvers. Figure 5.8 outlines the typical phases leaders go though as they transform from traditional to lean leadership.

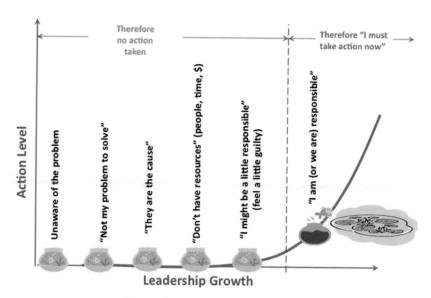

Figure 5.8: Leadership growth curve

Lean leadership requirements include the following:

1. Create a system that makes the waste visible, so that everyone can see it and appropriately focus improvement efforts.
2. Understand the truth (based on hard data) about the work by spending time in the gemba, observing each process before rendering a judgment on how to fix an issue. Leaders cannot understand the problem from the conference room or a private office.
3. Define and demand true success. Don't select improvement areas based on what you believe is possible. Improve based on what is necessary by virtue of the customers' requirements. The most innovative thinking is often driven by what was considered an "impossible" problem.
4. Act on problems right away; do not procrastinate.
5. Help the team solve problems in the gemba—ask "why" at least five times, and commit to understanding and solving the issues with the intent that they will never recur. This is root cause problem solving.
6. Relentlessly work with your team to identify and minimize all forms of waste and unnecessary variation.

As stated earlier, it is critical to identify and engage key leaders at the outset of the lean journey. Here are some tips on what it takes to be a great leader:

1. Be an excellent listener. This skill is especially important when reviewing process in the gemba (acute care wards, clinic, ORs, etc.). If process problems are observed, lean leaders should be curious about their cause and observe the issue carefully before giving an opinion on how to proceed. When thinking about how to work through process problems, remember the "Three Actual" rule. Go to the *actual place* where the issue is occurring, observe the *actual issue*, and talk to the *actual people* involved (don't forget to thank them for their input). After going through these steps, lean leaders work with their team to solve the problem at its root. Although this takes longer than

issuing an order with little data, the effect of solving a problem once and for all is worth the effort. There will be those who are skeptical of lean management. Leaders must listen carefully to their concerns, empathize with them, state the case for change, express confidence in the change, and demonstrate the vast opportunities for improvement.

2. Be an excellent communicator. Change is difficult for many people, and leaders must "connect the dots" for the organization, clearly communicating the case for a change and what that will entail. It must be emphasized that lean problem solving requires not only lean methods but a management system and a mindset (culture) change; it is not just another "project" or initiative. The quicker the organization understands that lean is not another project but is the way it does business, the easier it will be to engage the workforce.

3. Encourage and empower the people who work for you. This sounds cliché, but it is a powerful goal that successful leaders maintain. An example is a team implementing a fix to a process that the manager knows won't work. Instead of shooting the idea down, the leader lets them try it and learn from their experience (as long as it is low risk and patients are not negatively impacted). Lean systems are based on continuous improvement. If a team tries and fails, that's okay, as long as it learns from the experience and improves the solution on the next iteration. Lean leaders should work to identify and support emerging leaders in the organization. Early on, focus on the champions, not the naysayers, and praise each small, positive step along the way.

4. Leaders need to be humble students. Like formal schooling, lean is much more about learning than it is about teaching. Leaders need to understand that they potentially know a small percentage of the reality of a given problem. Before leaders give direction, they must "put their student hat on" and learn the facts of the issue (hard data) instead of going off of a gut feeling or anecdotes. They need to view all their work as experimental. If a directional change is called for, they should

not be afraid to change, even if it runs counter to directions they set earlier. They always encourage suggestions for change.

5. Leaders need to be relentless in working toward the ideal state—many times they stop themselves before they even try. Lean leaders know that they don't need all the answers to solve seemingly insurmountable problems. They peck away at them in an iterative fashion until the desired outcome is achieved. A "backward plan" strategy can be powerful. When taking on large issues, clarify the end goal, including the completion date, and work backward from the finish date to plan the project. In this way, a lean leader will specify what must be done and then create an iterative plan to accomplish the goal rather than become paralyzed by thinking he/she has no resources to apply to the issue. Lean problem solving is all about seeing opportunities, experimenting, failing at some, and continually improving. To quote Winston Churchill, "Success is going from failure to failure without losing enthusiasm."

6. Create a thinking shift. Executive and human resource alignment must change. When everyone is engaged in seeing and removing waste, the overall system improves. The single biggest roadblock to a successful, enterprise-wide lean implementation is reluctance to change. People may have been promoted to senior-level positions by acting in a traditional manner, and changing to another leadership paradigm goes against everything they have been rewarded for in the past. This is why successful lean implementation is more about transforming thinking than it is about implementing lean tools.

Engaging Senior Management

It has been our experience that engaging executives in a meaningful way is the biggest stumbling block for most lean transformations. This is problematic because the organization takes its cues from the behaviors of the senior executives. As each group works through the details of implementing lean systems in its area, it watches what the executive team is doing. If the executives lead by example (by going to the gemba and helping the frontline staff solve their issues), this will give the area teams the direction they need to proceed with challenging work. If the executive team does little to embrace the lean transformation by taking an active role, everyone quickly realizes that the effort is "just another top-down initiative" to weather until it dies. The executive team's sustained involvement in a lean transformation is the most important requirement for long-term success.

Typically, executives start their lean journey with strategy deployment—deciding on the big, important initiatives—and then aligning resources to meet those needs. Although this is important, it can feel a lot like the old work of setting direction and demanding results. The lean leadership approach is different, because it asks leaders (starting with executives) to be highly engaged in value added work. This can be done only by understanding the issues in the gemba that slow the transformation and relentlessly working to remove roadblocks. Strategies that are both realistic and strategically important are achieved only through understanding capabilities at the frontlines. To do that, the executive team needs to show its commitment to the coaching required to change from a more traditional, top-down model to one that emphasizes "servant leadership." (Figure 5.9)

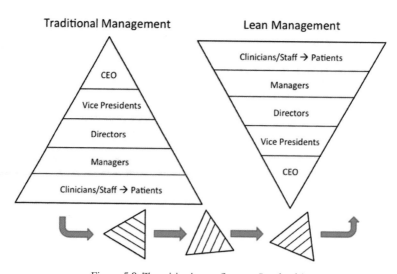

Figure 5.9: Transitioning to Servant Leadership

Switching to a servant leadership role from an order-giver role is a big challenge that must be overcome if the lean transformation is to be successful. We discuss this in following chapters, but for now, the important thing is to understand what a great lean leader is and to commit to becoming one.

Basic lean (better hockey) can be done without full engagement at all levels of leadership, but advanced lean (ballet) requires engagement from all leadership levels (executives to the frontline). We describe this change as a shift from managing by objectives to managing by process or servant leadership.

Changing the behaviors of the executive team is one of the most challenging aspects of a lean transformation. This is a paradox, because the executive team likely decided to pursue lean in the first place. The challenge does not stem from some issue inherent to the executives but rather because lean management systems require a mindset that is different from the traditional management by objective (MBO) system most executives practice. Typical MBO leadership is characterized by a strict focus on results, prioritization of projects over core workflows, little tolerance for failure, and the consequent devaluation of experimentation around process redesign. Other differences between lean management and traditional MBO management are shown in table 5.1.

Traditional Management	Lean Management
Focus on outcome ("get results")	Focus on standardized processes that get the desired outcome
Attaining goals trumps all else	Developing people has equal weight to goal attainment
Manage to industry benchmarks	Manage to customer requirements
Metrics visible to few	Metrics visible to all
Batch and retrospectively review results	Real time and prospective view of data/results
Management tells staff what to do	Management questions, challenges, coaches and offers help to staff
Manage from office	Manage in gemba
Problems are bad	Problems are treasures
What person produced the error?	What suboptimal work process(es) or system produced error
Autocratic, top-down problem solving	Guided, distributed, participative problem solving
Autocratic, top-down goal creation	Guided, distributed, participative goal creation
Organizational success attained by time-intensive analysis and design of "perfect fix"	Success through continuous, rapid, small, incremental improvements

Table 5.1: Traditional (MBO) Management compared to Lean
(Manage By Process) Management

Without a clear and unwavering vision for transformation, a focus on running the business in a fundamentally different way and transforming critical business units, MBO will persist, and the lean transformation will not occur. The result is lean techniques practiced in an MBO organization. It is not uncommon to see lean done "around" executives, particularly at level 2 (better hockey). In this setting, executives are the cheering section for the hockey game—they are supporters but not players. They unleash lean unto the frontline and give the team verbal support, resources, and adulation. They allow lean to "flourish" at the frontlines, reporting that "lean is an organically grown initiative."

If further executive development cannot be achieved, two problems will result. First, when lean is seen as an initiative and not how the organization intends to run business, potential late adopters will entrench in the old system, and the transformation may fail. Second, organizational alignment will not be maintained around the transformation, and conflicting strategic initiatives will encroach. The executive team needs to make lean a mandate and demand transformation of critical business units using the method (principally, the value stream view). They must transform themselves from spectators to humble students who no longer demand objectives (MBO) but demand and support outstanding processes created in partnership with the front line workers (servant leadership). This is a key difference with lean management as it engages the staff in solving *their* problems instead of the executives' problems. It also focuses on the key drivers (processes) that will give the improvement results needed. To quote Jim Womack, founder and senior advisor of the Lean Enterprise Institute, "If you work on the correct processes, the results will be correct. If you work on the wrong processes and the results are correct, someone is lying."

Lean goal setting is a highly participative catch-ball process in which top management proposes enterprise-wide goals that are vetted up and down the organization's chain of command. This goal-setting process is termed *hoshin kanri*. Hoshin kanri links the improvement activities of leaders and work groups at all levels so that they work toward common goals—ultimately the organization's true north. It gives visibility to individual and group accountabilities. In this way, goals are quantified, methods for achieving goals are clearly communicated, and roles and expectations are agreed upon before action is taken. Hoshin kanri provides a mechanism that enables all employees to understand how their personal goals directly relate to and impact the strategic goals of the organization.

Let's look at an example of how an organization can use hoshin kanri planning to set goals and develop a management by process or lean management system. A healthcare organization is beginning its lean transformation, and it determines that its annual quality goal will be a 20 percent reduction in quality defects. This goal is deployed throughout the organization, and the executive team receives input on how it can best be interpreted for all of the business units (clinical and nonclinical). For example, the intensive care units (ICUs) determine that their biggest quality defect is central line-associated blood stream infections (CLABSIs).

Once management agrees that this problem is aligned with the organization's overall quality goal, management should not blindly sit back and monitor the ICU's CLABSI results on a monthly, quarterly, or semiannual basis. Management should insist that the teams determine the processes or the drivers of CLABSIs, based on the best-known evidence. For CLABSIs, these drivers are sterile insertion technique, proper hand hygiene, sterile technique when accessing and de-accessing the line, and proper timing and technique for changing the central line's dressing.

With a management by process focus, the organization is focused on the aforementioned four drivers that are known to lead to CLABSIs. Processes are mapped, standards are set, staff and clinicians are trained on the new standards, processes are audited, the results are posted, and barriers to meeting the standardized processes are managed. With this type of alignment and laser focus on the CLABSI drivers (that is, focus from senior management down to the frontline workers), the outcome of fewer CLABSIs will be reliably and sustainably attained.

Creating an Engaged Workforce: Aligning Human Resources

Everyone needs to know that at its core, lean is a system that increases customer satisfaction and improves staff and corporate needs by reducing non-value added work. This is done by implementing standardized practices to make everyone's work as efficient as possible. These standard processes (called standardized work) must be constructed by the people who actually do the work, not external people who are unfamiliar with the processes. This ensures that the day-to-day realities of the workplace are taken into account and that ownership resides appropriately with those in the gemba.

All players in a lean transformation need to be engaged by drafting a true north statement that bridges the needs of the patients, staff, clinicians, and business. This will help pique the groups' interest in the work instead of seeing lean implementation as a distraction from their primary business. One must be relentless in getting cross-functional groups to work on the transformation at the outset. Each group must be represented by lean champions who can communicate the benefits of lean to their team. Champions are needed at all levels: physicians, nurses, staff, managers, and executives.

Once an improvement team is identified, it needs to be educated on the details of lean systems. Some of the best education at the beginning phase is to visit other organizations that are operating within a lean system at the enterprise level. Taking "study missions" to lean sites is a common approach, and the sooner this happens, the sooner that real gains can be realized.

If we look to the structures of ballet troupes, we can see many of the ingredients for successful operational teams in healthcare organizations:

1. Act as a team rather than as an individual (a "we" rather than a "me" mentality). In ballet, it's more important to be a great team member than it is to play as an individual contributor. Everyone knows that one great dancer does not make *Swan Lake*.
2. Have a well-thought-out plan and follow it. Every successful troupe needs a script so that the dancers work harmoniously on every move. The script for healthcare operations is standardized work.

3. Rely on great coaching. Every successful ballet troupe needs coaching to make small corrections as the dance is rehearsed. Coaching in an operational setting is called "visual control" and "management response."
4. Use a scoreboard to track progress. The scoreboard for a business is called a business plan; it tracks actual versus planned outcomes and highlights where help is needed to improve expected outcomes.

Engaging Physicians

A successful lean transformation, at all levels, requires engagement of all stakeholders. Physicians are no exception, because they are major stakeholders on the healthcare team. We have witnessed that a minority of physicians are early adopters or vehement objectors (bordering on frank obstructionists). Most are "on the sidelines," waiting and watching, curious but suspicious, often betting that the "how we will now run the business" mantra by administration will fade away (much like other "initiatives" that veteran physicians have lived through). They may cynically believe that lean is the latest cost-cutting program imported from another industry rather than a path to create value for their patients.

Most physicians don't readily see the link between the system of care (i.e., the processes that support patient care) and the content of care (the care itself that they provide). For instance, it has been shown that adverse patient outcomes are most often due to bad processes, not bad people[12]. With that in mind, why do physicians have trouble seeing the link between the process of care and the content of care? Conversely, why do lean leaders have trouble making this connection for physicians? What is it about the lean culture and language and the physician culture and language that promote this chasm? Undeniably, lean culture and physician culture are aligned in their missions: to provide the highest quality and safest outcomes for patients.

In this section, we define "lean culture" as the behaviors and expectations of nonphysician leaders of a lean transformation in any healthcare setting. How this supports or seemingly contradicts the "physician culture" was addressed in an outstanding webinar produced by the Healthcare Value Network.[13] Dr.

Mark Hallett, senior medical director at ThedaCare, a five-hospital community healthcare system in Appleton, Wisconsin, discussed the differences in lean and physician cultures that, if not understood and addressed, can lead to persistent non- or under-engagement of the physician workforce. The salient differences, based on Hallet's research and our own experiences, are summarized in table 5.2.

	Lean Culture	Physician Culture
Customer	Patient is customer	Elective care: patient is a customer Fiduciary care: patient is simply a patient
Responsibility and Liability	Trust processes and the people that influence the process	Processes don't get sued, physicians do based on their patient outcomes
Getting to root cause	Ask why five times	Ask who
Bias for action	Go slow to go fast	Quick, outcome oriented
Leadership	Humility based; typical hierarchy triangle flipped 180 degrees	All-knowing; work-arounds and fire-fighting rewarded Hierarchy rules
Language	Japanese and business terms based on systems thinking for process improvement	Medical terms based on systems thinking for patient diagnosis and treatment
Scientific Method	PDCA processes	PDCA clinical care
Patients' Journey	Inch deep, mile wide	Mile deep, inch wide
Defects	Not tolerated	Often taboo to discuss
Principal approach to care	Science of medicine	Art and science of medicine
Premise upon which to base care or improvement decisions	Data	Data

Table 5.2: Lean Culture Compared to Physician Culture

Understanding Cultural Differences

The first aspect to be addressed maps to the first level of our lean operations house: gaining organizational alignment as to who the customer is. The two aspects of this alignment are defining the customers and defining their requirements.

First, we must agree that the "customer" is the patient. This sounds simple, but to many physicians, it is anathema to how they have long been nurtured and rewarded in healthcare. Historically, the healthcare system was built around the physician as the customer, foremost serving his/her needs, which often are at odds with good patient service (e.g., build big waiting rooms so that patients can wait for the physician and the physician does not risk waiting for patients). Additionally, physicians who are expert at patient care have been promoted into administrative positions without adequate training and mentorship. Their influence over system-based processes can be misdirected, despite the best intentions. Physicians enjoy patient-care autonomy (to the extent that it makes sense for the diseases they treat), but this autonomy, when exercised for changing care processes, can result in batched processes, waste in the form of long patient wait times, and a host of other inefficiencies.

In a lean culture, the patient is the customer. Extending this thinking to the issue of service, the "customer is always right," and thus it is paramount to listen to the voice of the customer. In the physician culture, physicians may argue that the patients are the customer when they have a choice, as in an elective surgical procedure for which there is more than one physician and institution to choose. However, physicians have argued that once they need to deliver care in a fiduciary manner (such as when an unconscious trauma patient arrives in the ED), the patient is a patient and not a customer.

The customer is not always right in the eyes of the physician. Patients may desire treatments that are not beneficial to them. However, their voice must be heard, because they often want to be a part of the clinical care decision-making team, and they have observations about the processes (e.g., wait times, way finding, or customer service) as they interact with the healthcare system. By listening to them, improvements in care content, processes, and empathetic discussions create an optimal healing environment.

Perceptions around liability need to be understood. A basic tenet of the lean culture is to have trust in both the processes that drive outcomes and the people who influence those processes. If the processes (drivers) of a particular desired outcome are right, the outcome will be right. The lean culture sees the processes as vital to the outcome. However, healthcare is judged by many solely on its outcomes;

it is difficult for people to "see" the critical processes. In addition, physicians have argued that processes don't get sued; physicians do. Although this is true, if the drivers (both clinical and nonclinical) of a patient care outcome are optimized, the result will most likely be optimized, making the physicians and their personal "microbrand" or reputation much less likely to be compromised.

The historical context of root cause problem solving that physicians have been trained in needs to be understood. This is best illustrated by understanding the decades-old "morbidity and mortality conference." These conferences have been predicated on identifying a person (or persons) to blame for a bad patient outcome and shaming them into better behavior. The focus is on that small number of instances when "bad" people produce the bad outcome or falsely attributing a bad outcome to a person rather than the "system" that the person is working in. Issues of judgment, intelligence, and poor hierarchical understanding are exclusively highlighted in such conferences, often at the expense of understanding how the system (the processes) failed the physician and the patient. The focus is on the "who."

In contrast, the default position for blame for a bad outcome in a lean culture is on the "what"—the processes that influence the outcome—which is the definition of a just culture. In other words, a just culture holds people accountable for following safe practices or processes rather than punishing for errors. In the lean system, workers aim to create an open, fair learning culture that strives to continuously improve processes using PDCA. This is attained by continually asking "why" until the root cause is identified. To define a safe system for a patient-care process, workers need to manage behavioral choices.

We are happy to say that there has been a shift toward a just culture in the morbidity and mortality conferences and that modern professional practice evaluations, as well as focused professional practice evaluations for physicians, are using the tenets of a lean culture. In doing so, three principle behaviors need to be managed. The first is human error—inadvertently doing something other than what should be done. It is a slip, a lapse, a mistake. Humans are fallible, and errors will occur. Leaders should console the individual and employ countermeasures such as improved processes and training. This is an ideal time to improve processes using error-proofing methods (these will be discussed in chapters 9 and 10).

The second action is "at-risk behavior." These are behavioral choices that increase risk when risk is not recognized or is mistakenly believed to be justified. Leaders should coach the individual and employ countermeasures such as removing incentives for at-risk behavior, creating incentives for healthy behavior, and increasing situational awareness.

The third action is "reckless behavior." It happens with a minority of healthcare workers and is the most serious. It is a behavioral choice to consciously disregard a substantial and unjustifiable risk. Reckless behavior is the only time when some form of punishment is justified, and the countermeasure can be remedial or punitive action.

The lean and physician cultures often differ with respect to their bias for action. In a lean culture, it is often important to "go slow to go fast." An example is creating an A3 storyboard to solve an important cross-functional process problem. Creating an A3 can be tedious and time consuming, but a detailed problem definition and identifying the root cause can lead to a swift, focused action plan. This is often in contrast to physician problem solving; they can be impatient with processes and jump to solutions without getting to the root cause. Fortunately, this is not how physicians problem solve for direct patient-related problems. The key to closing this gap is to demonstrate the nearly identical nature of physician problem identification and solving through the traditional history, physical, supplementary testing, cognitive assembly of data, analysis of response, and adjustments to care plan and compare this to the lean problem solving through PDCA. The scientific method for lean and medical care is identical, and tension arises when the connections between the two are not explicitly called out. Both are steeped in PDCA. For physicians, PDCA loops are sometimes unconsciously based on pattern recognition and experience garnered over many years of patient care. This experience does not translate as readily to process problem solving, but it can be explained using terms that are familiar to physicians.

When including physicians in process problem solving, consider starting with "What is your hypothesis?" or "What could we measure that would tell us whether or not the experiment being proposed worked?" This is in contradistinction to the simple but culturally foreign question, "What problem are you trying to solve?" often posed by lean zealots.

The following is a quote from the Lean Enterprise Institute blog post by Dr. Jack Billi, associate dean and vice president of medical affairs at the University of Michigan:

> Physicians use scientific problem solving daily when they compare their patient's findings with known syndromes and diseases, to create a hypothesis about the patient's tentative diagnosis. They use root cause analysis in their "Impression," including alternative explanations ("The jaundice might be caused by biliary obstruction or a reaction to a nausea drug"), and in developing a **P**lan of care (countermeasures). The hypothesis is tested (**D**o) and revised by further diagnostic testing or by response to treatment, a form of **C**heck and **A**djust. No physician I know would consider treating or performing surgery on a patient he or she had not personally examined—"gone to the gemba," so to speak. It's just not acceptable.[14]

Billi is alluding to the need for data to drive decision-making. Nothing speaks more clearly and loudly to physicians than accurate data—it is the basis for a large part of their clinical decision-making. Data will go a long way to helping them understand the gaps in patient care processes, thus garnering their engagement and assistance. To quote W. Edwards Deming, father of PDCA, "In God we trust; all others bring data."

A lean culture views leadership as an exercise in humility. Lean leaders are not expected to be all-knowing, and they recognize that frontline workers know the problems intimately. The role of leadership is to serve, coach, and support the frontline. Hierarchy is important only in that the typical hierarchical management triangle needs to be turned 180 degrees, putting the frontline on the top and management on the bottom. However, in the physician culture, hierarchy is important. The senior physician has experience and knowledge for patient care that others can attain only after years of practice. Because physicians are solution oriented, their ascension in seniority and leadership is garnered by quick solutions, often attained by making "diving catches," firefighting, and coming up with work-arounds and quick fixes. This culture rewards continuous improvising for care processes, not continuous improvement.

In the same way that a physician's language can be foreign to nonphysicians, a lean culture is steeped in Japanese and business terms. These terms can be confusing (or even regarded as insulting) to physicians such that the language itself becomes a barrier to adoption. This is not unique to physicians, and it applies to all healthcare workers who are learning lean systems. Physicians try to speak to their patients in a language that is understandable, and lean leaders need to do the same for people who are not familiar with their terms. Table 5.3 gives examples of common lean terms and their translation into terms that resonate with physician and other direct care providers.

LEAN TERM	TRANSLATION
Value Stream	Care Pathway
Standard Work	Leading Practice
Waste	Inefficiency
Defect	Error that reaches patient
Gemba	Clinic, operating room, ward
A3/PDCA	Scientific method
Overproduction	Prep for patients who don't show
Inventory	Patients waiting, backlog of supplies or appointments

Table 5.3: Deciphering Lean Terms for Physicians

The patient's journey is viewed with a different lens in the lean culture versus the physician culture. Physicians principally work in a silo; their interactions with their patients are an "inch wide and a mile deep." Although healthcare is increasingly complex and a patient's care relies on teamwork among many practitioners, practitioners view their role in the patient's journey as narrow. Conversely, lean management looks at the patient in the same way that patients view their own navigation through the healthcare system: in a longitudinal fashion (the value stream view). Patients stream through the system by intersecting with many silos including physicians, nursing, and information technology experts. The processes that intersect these silos often produce a suboptimal patient experience. This does not mean that physicians should not demand and retain deep content expertise in their silo. It means that they need to understand how decisions made in one silo may or may not affect another and ultimately the patient. It is these "between-silo" processes that are often broken or misaligned and where healthcare can use assistance from physicians.

Lean aims for zero quality defects. Nothing else is tolerated. As an example, high-reliable industries such as nuclear power and commercial aviation operate at around a six sigma defect ratio (3.4 defects per million events). Healthcare is presently around two to three sigma for defects. We tolerate defective processes. We employ work-arounds and quick fixes but rarely solve problems at their root or, better yet, by mistake proofing systems. We speculate that this is, in part, due to the sentiment that defects or mistakes in the physician culture are taboo. Physicians are held to standards that approach infallibility by society, and they hold themselves to those unattainable standards. We strive for perfection with patient care but don't apply the same rigor to process problem solving.

Finally, the practice of medicine is steeped in the "solitary artisan" culture. It has evolved from a pure practice of an "art" to one that requires a combination of artistic cognitive assimilation of data based on pattern recognition, experiential learning, and evidence-based methods. However, the physician culture is often resistant to lean systems, because the lean culture places emphasis on the science of medicine by espousing clinical standardized work—often misinterpreted by physicians as "cookbook medicine." As mentioned earlier, lean vocabulary is obscure to newcomers, and the term "standardized work," if not properly explained, may be off-putting for physicians. Physicians value using their critical thinking skills in service to their patients. They don't want to practice cookbook medicine or have someone outside of the profession tell them how to best care for their patients.

If standardized work is explained to physicians as the "best way we (the collective evidence base) know now to practice and to reliably produce desired results," resistance will melt away. Standardized work should be viewed as how we've designed our work to *consistently* deliver safe, effective care. In addition, standardized work makes it possible for physicians to apply their creativity to improve work methods. Without standardized work, how would anyone know if a change is actually an improvement? The sanctity of the physicians' creativity and experience in solving patient problems is preserved. Clinical standardized work (e.g., clinical pathways) aim to standardize as much as possible and let patient variation be the only variation in the system. The difficult, rare, odd patient problem is one that requires the artistic side of the physician to come up with a solution.

There is no one prescription for helping physicians understand and engage in lean practices. Understanding the physician culture in the context of lean culture and language is key, and actively working to close real or perceived gaps is a must. One must also recognize that healthcare organizations have subcultures of influencers (e.g., nurses and physicians), some with formal or informal influence outside traditional lines of organizational authority. Regardless of whether you are a lean leader or a physician learning about lean, both factions need to listen to the voice of the patient. What does the patient want? How can I (the physician) work within the bigger "system" to help deliver what patients want? Who can support me in this work?

One must emphasize to physicians that lean is first and foremost about quality and safety. Also, if successfully implemented, it will give the providers more time. This is time that physicians can spend with patients, time they can be helping with improvement events, and time that allows them to do research, teach, or get home at a reasonable hour. It is aimed at leveling the workload and reducing staff and physician overburden. Patient access to see physicians and use the healthcare system's services is augmented; more patients can be seen in a clinic, more can access the ORs, and fewer will wait in long queues for service.

Priming the Pump: Key Resources Needed for a Lean Transformation

Performance Improvement (PI) Team

Because the entire enterprise will be transformed, a multipronged approach to training is needed. This will include didactic training in a classroom setting, touring other lean organizations, and attending lean conferences, as well as individual study (some excellent references are available in the bibliography at the end of this book).

Another important way to educate an organization is by having a strong, house-wide communication plan, which should include reports at the end of lean events, as well as weekly and monthly updates on the organization's progress. Most importantly, the teams doing the actual improvement work in the gemba will need help. These duties usually fall under the purview of the "performance improvement (PI) team." It goes by many names—kaizen promotions office (KPO), lean resource office (LRO), continuous improvement team (CIT), etc.—but its core responsibility is to act as a catalyst for the organization's lean transformation. Typically, this group consists of lean coaches who often work with external lean *senseis* for guidance. The key attributes of this team are as follows:

1. Deep understanding of lean methodologies
2. Excellent facilitator skills (people skills)
3. Excellent project management skills
4. Excellent change management skills; they often partner with organizational development experts in the human resources department
5. Willingness to get involved with the work in the gemba; be present, be visible, be credible; the famous statement "if the student isn't learning, the teacher isn't teaching" must be at the forefront of the PI coach's mind
6. Willingness to help adjudicate the tension between vertically oriented, silo (authority-based) problem solving versus horizontally oriented, patient flow (responsibility-based) problem solving

As these points show, the PI team is much more than a project management team. Even though its numbers are typically relatively small (approximately one PI coach for one hundred to two hundred staff), it is critical that the team feels responsible for ensuring that its improvement work results in real gains. It does this by carefully selecting areas that have management teams that can succeed with lean transformations, as well as by helping to troubleshoot the new processes once they are in place.

Continuing Education and Engagement

Continuing education and engagement in and out of the gemba is required from everyone from the senior management to the frontline staff. Figure 5.10 compares optimal engagement to what typically happens. Keeping everyone engaged throughout the lean transformation is critical.

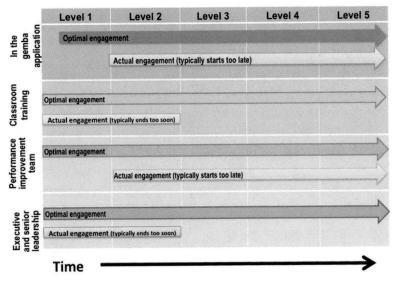

Figure 5.10: Optimal vs. Typical lean engagement

Local Problem Solving Teams

Root cause problem solving, countermeasure implementation, and designing new standards are the key skills that an organization needs to sharpen as

109

it progresses in its lean journey. Clinical quality and safety issues (e.g., patient hand-offs, catheter infections), regulatory issues (equipment as fire hazards in walkways), and a myriad of nonclinical problems (excessive wait times in clinic) will demand attention above and beyond applying quick countermeasures. Countermeasures, in this instance, refers to the daily work-arounds and firefighting to keep patient flow or nonclinical business flow proceeding. These quick, temporary, and necessary "fixes" are the job of middle management. However, mechanisms to record and prioritize these problems should be in place so that they do not happen again.

The work of the lean problem-solving team is root cause problem solving expertise. There must be time for this work, and it must be a part of their job (e.g., nurse manager), or there must be separate remuneration for their time (e.g., medical direction dollars for physicians). Team members aside from nurses and physicians include experts from the PI department, the clinical quality department, and support services as needed (e.g., IT, analytics, and engineering). Undying support by the hospital's executive team is paramount to their success. The executive team must be made aware of issues that cannot be resolved locally and then help remove barriers so that the team can take problem solving to its completion. These teams are trained together by solving an actual problem using A3 thinking based on John Shook's book, *Managing to Learn*,[15] and the eight-step problem solving developed at Toyota depicted in figure 5.11.[16]

Once trained, the team meets regularly, during stand-up meetings in the gemba or in a conference room, to review progress and priorities. They are supported by a daily management system that provides a clear path for barrier escalation (seeking help from the organization to overcome the barriers impeding problem solving that cannot be solved by the local team) and ways to make the work visible. The teams should share lessons learned and results both locally and with the broader healthcare community. It is beneficial that they publish their work or share via healthcare improvement blogs (e.g., Lean Post of the Lean Enterprise Institute) or via national collaboratives such as California Perinatal Quality Collaborative, Vermont Oxford Network, Lean Enterprise Institute, and the Healthcare Value Network.

Problem Solving Steps		Processes for each step
P	1. Clarify the problem.	1. Identify the ultimate goal. 2. Identify the ideal target condition. 3. Identify the gap.
	2. Break down the problem.	1. Break down the problem. 2. Select the specific problem to solve. 3. Specify the point of cause (go and see).
	3. Set aim/target.	1. Commit. 2. Set a measurable, concrete, challenging target/aim.
	4. Perform root cause analysis.	1. Without preconception, consider as many potential causes as possible. 2. Based on facts gathered by going and seeing, keep asking "why?" 3. Specify the root cause.
	5. Develop countermeasures.	1. Develop as many as possible. 2. Narrow them down to the most practical and effective. 3. Build consensus with others. 4. Create a clear and detailed action plan.
D	6. See countermeasures through.	1. Quickly and as a team, implement countermeasures. 2. Share progress by following, reporting, informing, and consulting communication practices. 3. Never give up, and proceed to the next step quickly.
C	7. Monitor results and process.	1. Evaluate the overall results and the processes used; share the evaluation with involved team members. 2. Evaluate from three viewpoints: patient (customer), organization, yours. 3. Understand factors behind success or failure (learn).
A	8. Standardize successful processes.	1. Structure the successful process (standardize). 2. Share the new precedent through horizontal deployment. 3. Start the next the round of incremental improvement.

Figure 5.11: Toyota's 8-Step Structured Problem Solving

In lean parlance, these teams are called *kaizen* operations teams (KOTs), moonshine teams, or resource teams. Interestingly, experts from the clinical quality world designed such a team, called the local improvement team (LIT), to solve quality and safety problems long before lean became popular in healthcare. The LIT is based on the "Clinical Microsystems" improvement model originally crafted by Dartmouth University.[17] It was intended to prioritize and develop standards for complex clinical quality problem solving. The LIT is a permanent, multidisciplinary team that is trained in improvement methodologies that assist the local management dyad (patient care manager and medical director) in delivering support to the frontline to produce reliably high quality outcomes for patients.

Dr. Paul Sharek, medical director of quality at the Lucile Packard Children's Hospital at Stanford (LPCH) embraced this concept soon after its conceptualization. His forward thinking brought the LIT concept to LPCH many years ahead of the organization's lean journey. Originally created in high-risk areas such as ICUs with a somewhat narrow scope (e.g., central line infections, as one example), Sharek's LIT work at LPCH is now a critical component of the Packard Quality Management System (the name for LPCH's lean operating system). LITs are now in place throughout the organization; they support clinical service lines (value streams) and shared services such as ICUs, ambulatory clinics, and perioperative services. They serve a long-term process improvement function in their areas. They inform goal deployment, complex problem solving, and setting new standards using a variety of lean tools, and they develop clinical standardized work, also known as care pathways.

How does this look in practice? Figure 5.12 depicts the LITs role in a lean system. The circles in the middle can be viewed as the two wheels of an "improvement bicycle." The front wheel of the bicycle depicts the frontline workers performing their daily work and area management managing to the unit's standards in a **S**tandardize, **D**o, **C**heck, **A**djust manner. Complex problems and the organization's annual core goals are dealt with by the back wheel of the bicycle in a **P**lan, **D**o, **C**heck, **A**djust (PDCA) manner.

As an example, a unit may have noticed a sustained spike in central venous catheter infections. Using any number of problem-solving techniques such as A3, rapid process improvement events, or 3P workshops, the LIT designs the new standards (countermeasures) that will be tested by the front wheel (frontline workers and local management).

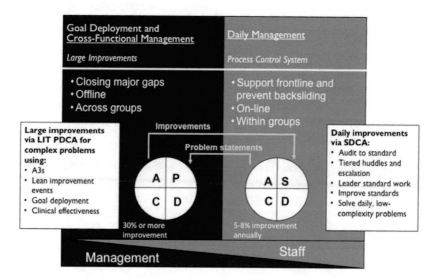

Figure 5.12: The two wheels of the continuous improvement bicycle

There can be an ad hoc or short-term nature to this type of problem solving. An example of this is in the perioperative area at Lucile Packard Children's Hospital. This area, operating at level 4, demands daily problem resolution, because it is operating against a certain cadence and continually trying to level the system. Although the organization started a series of week-long kaizen events a few years ago, the present system only occasionally requires that type of effort, often only for large, cross-functional problems. However, daily problems are dealt with by management and a PI expert who is assigned to the area. The PI expert works in the area every day with the staff and builds the gadgets/forms that the team doesn't have the time or expertise to do. These tasks include typing standardized work, ordering and building level-loading boxes, and implementing andon systems.

Create a Calendar

As a critical first step, the executive and management teams should create a calendar that allows the organization to do improvement work and oversight. A good place to start is creating a meeting-free zone; this is a time on a specific day (or every day) when no cross-functional meetings can occur so that work in the gemba can take place. Meetings in the gemba are allowed during this time because the spirit of this protected time is to not take area managers away from the gemba by virtue of cross-functional meetings (e.g., a multidisciplinary steering committee led by the information technology team). Synchronize this time with everyone's calendar so that others don't try to schedule meetings that you cannot attend.

Another way to institute meeting-free time is to create a theme for days of the week (Table 5.4). This works particularly well for diverse groups; everyone knows what is and is not allowed on a given day.

	Work with your team day	Cross-functional day	Work with your team day	Cross-functional day	Work with your team day
	Monday	**Tuesday**	**Wednesday**	**Thursday**	**Friday**
7:00					
8:00					
9:00					
10:00					
11:00			Meeting-free zone		
12:00					
13:00					
14:00					
15:00					
16:00					
17:00					
18:00					

Table 5.4: Daily calendar

How to Get Started

Getting a lean transformation to occur at the enterprise level will take more than reading a book and following the rules it prescribes. Lean will need to be seen as the solution to the pressing issues that your enterprise faces. It must be important enough to overcome the hardship of getting the entire organization to act differently.

To get started, your lean journey will need the following things:

1) Acquire lean support (e.g., a sensei). This is a critical first step in any lean transformation and is especially important in advanced lean. Shop around, because not all lean experts are created equal. You will want experts who have a lot of experience transforming and operating lean enterprises from level 1 to level 5. They need to be able to communicate effectively to your team at all levels—"it's no good being

the smartest book on the shelf if no one reads you." Good lean senseis should be a bit pushy, because their job is to get the team to a place that would not have been possible without their help. Don't be afraid to ask for references. Even better, visit a few sites that the sensei has helped transform.

2) Assemble the team. You must have senior leadership participation from the start. This includes executives as well as nursing and physician leadership. It's not necessary for this group to be lean zealots, but they must be open to working together to improve all three legs of the business system (patients, staff, organization). Over time, their roles will change to look like Table 5.5.

Lean operational executive and medical leaders:
- Champion the transformation by following their daily standardized work.
- Have a deep understanding of the improvement work
- Are responsible for removing barriers that the team cannot solve

---

Table 5.5: Core Leadership Responsibilities

An important thing to remember when working with senior leaders is that they are learning along with the organization. Traditionally, senior leaders had to "know the answers" to the difficult problems—that's how they were promoted. In an advanced lean transformation, they are asked to change from being *order givers* to being *students and enablers* of the frontline workers. This is a big change for the senior leadership team, and it will not be an easy one. Patience is required on everyone's part as the senior team improves its lean leadership skills.

3) Clearly state the current problems with the system. Your statement should include patient issues (cost, quality, access, and empathy), corporate issues (volume, pricing, costs, and profits), and staff issues (work hours, management support, engagement, and pay levels). Once you have this statement, you need agreement on where to begin. It's critical that you pick the most pressing issues. Picking the "must do, can't fail" issues as the starting point for an advanced lean transformation may seem counterintuitive. Many groups choose to focus on less critical goals at the start so that they can learn in an easier setting. The problem with this approach is that it won't force senior leaders to change their management behaviors anytime soon. Remember that lean is not as much about the end results as it is about building the processes and developing the people to be able to deliver the end results. Get the leaders at all levels thinking and acting correctly as soon as possible. Only the issues of the highest priority will force them to focus on acting differently.

4) Define the current state of each critical issue. One example is shown in Table 5.6.

The critical issues from an outpatient clinic:
• Patient – Access time too long
• Staff – Staff is unengaged
• Corporation – Profit is too low

Table 5.6: Defining the Problem(s)

Now that the issues have been defined, it is time to better understand their condition. For example, if patient-access time for a clinic is too long, the first question is, "How long is it?" This will inevitably bring up questions of what is in and out of scope. Will waiting room time be counted, or is it just the time from the patient requesting a service to seeing a provider? These questions have to be answered so that the current state can be mapped (Figure 5.13). Similarly, staff engagement and corporate profit will need to be defined and their current state well understood, preferably with hard numbers, so that a baseline can be created.

Current state of the outpatient clinic
- Current patient wait times by service
  - ENT = 7.5 days
  - Ortho = 15.4 days
  - Gen = 34.2 days
  - Urology = 3.4 days
- Staff engagement
  - Staff-led improvements: improvements / week / team member = 0.15
  - Staff absenteeism: hours / week / team member = 3.2
- Current profit margin by service
  - ENT = +5.4%
  - Ortho = -1.2%
  - Gen = -3.4%
  - Urology = +12.3%

Figure 5.13: Current state data

5) Clearly state success against the critical issues. Now that the current state is known, describe what "success" would be or what the goal is for each critical measure (Figure 5.14).

Future state
- Goal for patient wait times by service
  - ENT = 1.5 days
  - Ortho = 5.0 days
  - Gen = 7.0 days
  - Urology = 3.4 days
- Goal for staff engagement
  - Staff-led improvements: improvements / week / team member = 1.0
  - Unplanned staff absenteeism: hours / week / team member = 0.5
- Goal for profit margin by service
  - ENT = +10.0%
  - Ortho = +7.0%
  - Gen = +5.0%
  - Urology = +12.3%

Figure 5.14: Future state goal

6) Assign senior leadership team as owners, and pick project teams. Once the current state and goals have been established, assign senior ownership and build sub-teams around each critical issue (Figure 5.15). In our example, project teams would be led by senior leaders. The access team might be led by the chief operating officer (COO) and the chief medical officer (CMO). The staff engagement team might be led by the vice president of human resources and the chief nursing officer (CNO). The profit goal team might be led by the chief financial officer (CFO) and the medical director or service chief of each clinical service. This may sound like a lot of overhead, but remember that these are the most pressing needs of the organization and that the goal is to create lean leaders who will coach the organization into a new way of acting.

Leadership team:
- Includes senior leaders, key members of the medical and operations leadership team
- Includes key support leaders (e.g., material, facilities)
- Responsible for spending the time it takes to thoroughly understand. Goes and sees the progress in the workplace and serves as mentors by doing A3s with the team.
- Responsible for solving cross-functional problems and ensuring the project's success

Project team
- Includes operations managers, lean resources, and data specialists
- Includes (part time): lean coach, communication specialist, IT resource, supply resource, key stakeholders, and potentially other functional support
- Responsible for building, implementing, and sustaining all new processes throughout the area

Figure 5.15: Teams and Their Roles

7) Build a document called an A3, which captures the problem statement, current state, and goals as depicted in Figure 5.16.

Problem statement:
Patient access time is too long

Proposed changes:

Current state:
Current patient wait times by service
- ENT = 7.5 days
- Ortho = 15.4 days
- Gen = 34.2 days
- Urology = 3.4 days

Plan:

Goal:
Goal for patient wait times by service
- ENT = 1.5 days
- Ortho = 5.0 days
- Gen = 7.5 days
- Urology = 3.4 days

Root-cause analysis:

Follow-up & measures:

Figure 5.16: A3 Problem Solving Template/Storyboard

8) Understand the causes of suboptimal performance. This can be done only by seeing the actual issues in the actual workplace and talking to the actual people who are experiencing the problems. These issues should be recorded and reported to the larger group by the senior leadership owner (executives and/or medical leaders). Traditionally, a fishbone diagram is used to group the issues into headings such as methods, equipment, staff, and supplies (Figure 5.17).

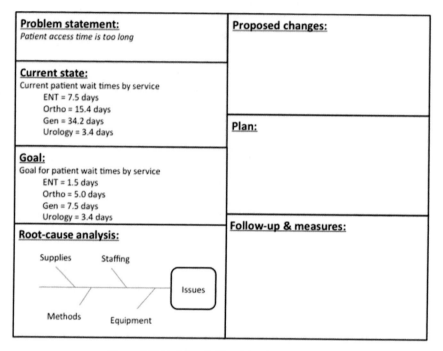

Figure 5.17: Left hand side of the A3 is complete

9) Now that the problem and goals are understood (the left side of the A3), solve the issues (right side of the A3) by applying an advanced lean operating system, covered in subsequent chapters.

CHAPTER 6

Level 2—Operational Stability

	No Waiting		Management System / People Development		Quality First	
Level 5 (optimize)	• Innovation to improve access, cost, empathy		• Refine leadership's & workforce's PDCA skills • Refine strategy deployment		• Innovation to improve quality / safety • Verify at the source	
Level 4 (takt environment)	• Set staff cycle times • Staff Standardized Work • Clinical standardized work		• Manage to standardized work & level flow • Immediate andon response		• Use andon for process stop to meet the standard • Successive check	
Level 3 (match capacity to demand)	Detail patient flow & lead times	Level loading	• Workflow control • Control process variation	Staff to demand	Understand cadence (takt)	
Level 2 (Stability)	• Establish flow • Initiate clinical std work	Quality & service stds.	Visual management and problem solving	Success metrics	Methods, Equipment, Staffing, Supplies (MESS) + 5S	
Level 1 (Foundation)	Leader engagement	Customer = patient	Shared values		Value stream thinking	

House roof: Extraordinary Patient Care — Highest Quality, Safety and Empathy; Easiest and Timely Access and Lowest Cost

Our discussion of level 1 stressed the need to educate the organization about aligning around patient flow. This included setting the vision for the organization's transformation and building the support structures to enable it. At level 2, the organization will develop basic operational stability. Operational stability is achieved by ensuring that all resources are available when needed and that they function reliably. Readily available supplies, scheduling, equipment, staffing, information, workplace orderliness, and reliable methods are examples of critical elements that need to be in order before moving to the next level. Inconsistencies in things such as information or supplies will make consistent workflows impossible because staff members will have to go out of their way to make up for the system's deficiencies. For example, a study of our inpatient units showed that nurses were spending up to 20 percent of their days looking for supplies.

In our hockey-to-ballet analogy, attaining operational stability is analogous to playing better hockey but setting the stage for ballet. This is the level where, in addition to achieving workplace stability, staff engagement and foundational lean training are put to the test. The enhanced lean knowledge garnered at this stage comes from learning by doing as opposed to the learning at level 1, which is largely done didactically.

The Concept of Flow

Flow is not just a lean term; it is the basis for creating and supporting the lean operating system.

Flow can be best described as follows. A patient requests service (care) from the healthcare system. A system with perfect flow responds by delivering care immediately (no waiting by the staff delivering the care or the patient receiving the care), with perfect quality, in the ideal healing environment (empathetic, mission-driven staff and clinicians), and using the fewest necessary resources (cost). Stated another way, a lean operating system ensures perfect patient flow by creating perfect processes designed to serve patients in a *continuously and uninterrupted* fashion across the continuum of care (from entry to exit of the system), creating value for the patient according to what the patient values and needs. It provides the highest quality and safest care that is based on the best scientific evidence and administered correctly the first time with no rework or complications. Care is provided with no waiting at a cost that doesn't deter patients or their insurance providers from using the particular healthcare system. Unless otherwise stated, the term "healthcare system" is used in this book to mean any type of integrated or stand-alone hospital or outpatient facility (private physician office, clinic, rehabilitation facility, subacute facility, surgery center).

It is critical to understand, from a pragmatic point of view, what flow looks like for patients. To do this, we use examples that demonstrate perfect, single-patient flow and what flow looks like when multiple patients request service.

Let's first use an example outside of healthcare: the blacksmith. A blacksmith's job is part transformation. Once the metal is maximally heated in the kiln, the blacksmith immediately goes to work and does not stop molding the metal until the product is finished. He never puts the metal down, because it needs to be shaped while it is hot. There is neither waiting nor wasted movement. The result is a continuous flow of material and process—this is a lean system at its most basic.

An equivalent single-patient example is the interplay between a surgeon and the assistant who hands the surgeon the instruments (the scrub technician or scrub nurse). All the materials needed are planned and meticulously distributed within arm's reach on the assistant's table. The surgeon continuously performs the procedure by being handed instruments without unnecessary movements by the surgeon or the assistant; this is repeated until the procedure is completed—thus, there is a continuous flow. This is an example of optimal patient and staff flow as well as supply and equipment flow.

A final example of excellent single-patient flow is when one patient comes to see a physician in an outpatient office. The patient enters the office and is immediately placed in an examination room. After the nurse records vital information, the physician enters the room and performs the indicated service using all the time necessary to connect with the patient and deliver the indicated care and teaching. Perfect care is administered without interruption or waiting.

These examples show that there is more than one flow to consider when invoking perfect patient flow. Aside from patient and supply/equipment flow, there is also "information flow" to consider. When all the necessary paperwork is filled out in advance of a patient's visit and no time is wasted in a waiting room, this exemplifies perfect information flow.

These examples demonstrate single patient/supplies/information flow—a basic lean system—optimized for a *single* patient. If multiple patients have identical clinical needs, and they access the system at the same time, and they require the same duration of service, the system would only need to increase the number of providers to meet the demand. However, this simplistic system is not realistic for any type of healthcare organization. Typically, patients demand care at different times of the day, with different levels of care and expertise, and with differing durations. This requires creating an advanced lean system designed for continuous flow in response to the cadence of demand by its heterogeneous cohort of patients, again with perfect quality, timeliness, and low cost. This type of system requires matching capacity to demand, creating standardized work for the staff and clinicians that does not over-burden them, and continuous elimination of wasteful processes.

Understanding an organization's flows requires mapping how patients move through the inpatient service lines and/or outpatient clinics. This value stream mapping should be understood and managed at the start of an organization's lean journey. However, patient flow will be characterized by constant, unanticipated stops and starts (like hockey) in a system that is replete with waste. High quality, timeliness, and cost effectiveness will not be *consistently and reliably* attained.

Once an organization is using a lean operating system to manage its patient flows, the system should use the creative talents of its staff and clinicians to continuously improve standardized processes, information, supplies, and equipment to reach higher levels of quality, timeliness, and cost reduction. All these are matched to the cadence of patient demand (like ballet). The result is a system that confers the best possible staff and patient experience at the lowest possible cost.

Area Readiness

"Area readiness" means checking for operational stability. The check is an audit, often performed by area management at the start and end of a shift. The audits ensure that an area can do repeatable work: the same work process in the same sequence, every time. Critical aspects of readiness include the following:

1. A workplace that makes readiness apparent at a glance
2. An area replete with supplies and equipment at the point of use
3. Ensured quality of supplies, equipment, information, and communication (e.g., expired supplies or inoperable equipment are removed)
4. Co-location of staff, supplies, and equipment for improved communication and decreased walking and waiting

MESS and 5S

The factors that affect any area's operational stability are MESS and workplace organization achieved through "sort, simplify, sweep, standardize, and sustain," also known as 5S. If any MESS items are supplied inconsistently at the workplace or their quality is unreliable, repeatable work will not be possible.

A unit's visibility board (Figure 6.1) shows its daily MESS status. The MESS headings are in the left column, and the work areas leaders are shown across the top, one per column. The red dots indicate that the area's MESS standards were not met at the start of the shift, and the reasons for not meeting the standards are written in the far right column.

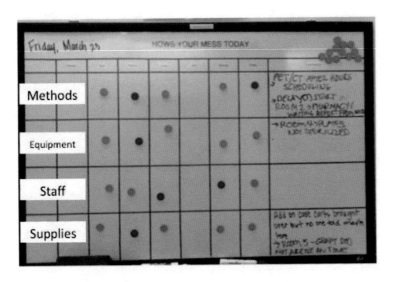

Figure 6.1: Methods, Equipment, Staffing, Supplies (MESS) readiness board

The Method Component of MESS

Methods outline how work can be done in an area with the highest efficiency and quality. Such methods are the reliable method or standards. Examples include how patients should be scheduled for appointments, how paperwork should be filled out in the admitting process, how clinicians and staff should perform proper hand hygiene, and how leaders should manage their areas. Notice the word "should" in every instance. In reality, most methods are not consistently followed, and because the goal is to create repeatable work sequences, it is critical to install consistent operating methods.

A single person's part of a method is a "work sequence." In a healthcare setting, lean methods are established by outlining work in a way that serves patient flow with the highest quality. This requires testing the method, documenting the best practice, building the work sequence into each staff person's daily routine, educating the work force on the sequence, and monitoring so that the sequence is followed correctly.

It is important that *all* work sequences have "quality gates"—process steps that must be performed in order for a patient to move to the next care process (Figure 6.2). For example, the World Health Organization (WHO) preoperative checklist (WHO Part 1) must be completed in its entirety for the patient to be moved into the OR, and a second checklist (WHO Part 2) must be completed prior to prepping and draping the patient for surgery.[18]

Surgery method with WHO checklist quality gates built-in

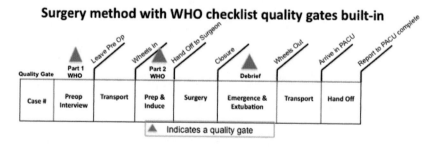

Figure 6.2: Quality gate example

Some methods are simple and consist only of one person's work sequence, such as how to perform proper hand hygiene (Figure 6.3), as proposed by the World Health Organization. In this example, the ability of a clinician to enter a patient's room for an examination—a quality gate—would depend on the clinician performing hand hygiene using the correct materials (cleanser) and sequence.

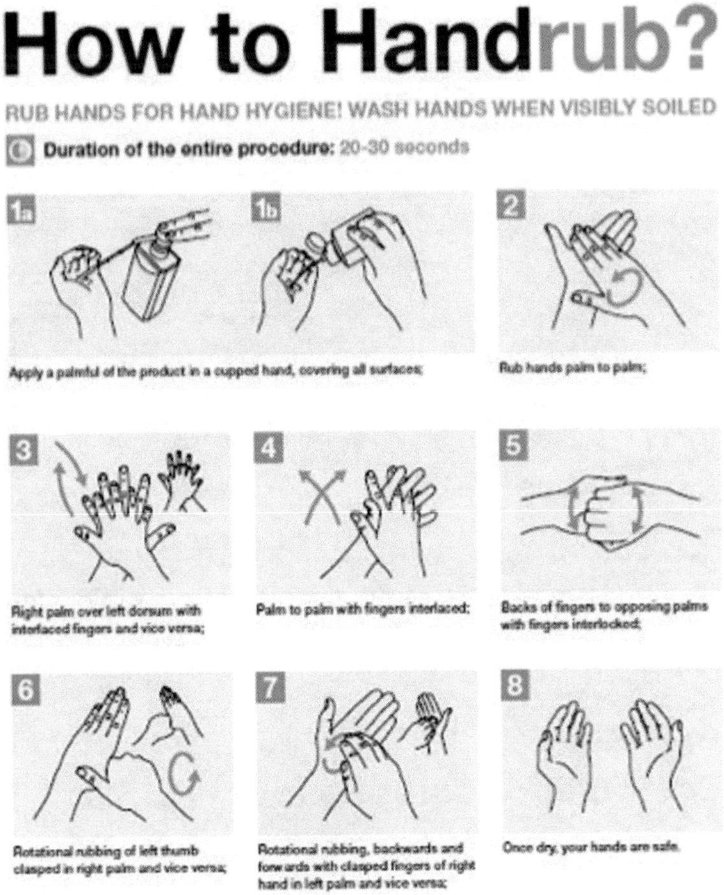

How to Handrub?

RUB HANDS FOR HAND HYGIENE! WASH HANDS WHEN VISIBLY SOILED

Ⓒ Duration of the entire procedure: 20-30 seconds

Apply a palmful of the product in a cupped hand, covering all surfaces;

Rub hands palm to palm;

Right palm over left dorsum with interlaced fingers and vice versa;

Palm to palm with fingers interlaced;

Backs of fingers to opposing palms with fingers interlocked;

Rotational rubbing of left thumb clasped in right palm and vice versa;

Rotational rubbing, backwards and forwards with clasped fingers of right hand in left palm and vice versa;

Once dry, your hands are safe.

Figure 6.3: Standard method for hand hygiene

Other methods are more complex, because they require multiple people with individual work sequences to complete them. The patient discharge method is a good example. On an obstetrics ward, many individuals impact the discharge of a baby and mother, and all caregivers have their own work sequence to support optimal patient flow, which is composed of a sequence of tasks. A work sequence for one event, transportation from the patient room to the car, is detailed in figure 6.4.

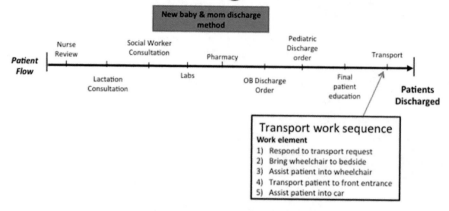

Figure 6.4: Work sequence for transport

Stable methods are not just for clinicians and staff; management also needs to consistently support the methods that best support patient flow. It is important to start with the process needs of the area and build the manager's daily schedule to support those processes.

The Equipment Component of MESS

Equipment that is missing, not easily found, dirty, or faulty can create workplace instability. From surgical tables that don't function correctly to intravenous pumps that are unavailable when needed, the availability of high-functioning equipment is critical to lean workflows.

Unlike supplies, equipment is generally reused, and so it needs to be cleaned, recalibrated, repaired, and stored so that it is ready for its next use. Good examples of reaching operational stability with equipment include the following:

1. Create a visual equipment readiness card; the status of the equipment can be noted at a glance (Figure 6.5).

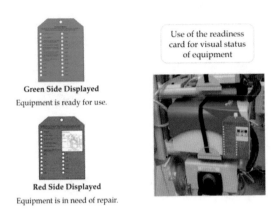

Use of the readiness card for visual status of equipment

Green Side Displayed
Equipment is ready for use.

Red Side Displayed
Equipment is in need of repair.

Figure 6.5: Equipment readiness cards

2. Create a special area for equipment in need of maintenance so that it is not put with functional equipment (Figure 6.6).

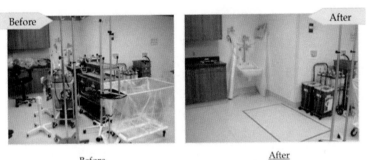

Before

After

No standard location for equipment in need of repair.

Space has been created for failed equipment storage consistent with 5S.

Figure 6.6: Equipment needing maintenance area

3. Like all other elements of operational stability, daily management is the key. Start by scheduling and performing preventive maintenance on equipment, and track the frequency of equipment failures. If equipment continues to show signs of failure, managers

129

need to work with their teams to determine what needs to be changed. In the following example, perhaps the frequency of maintenance on the low pressure system should be increased on the anesthesia machine to more than once per year, given the number of failures (Table 6.1).

Anesthesia Machine:	# of failures
Low pressure system leaks	73
Control panel wont stay seated	6
Flow sensor errors	5
O2 cell problems	7
Miscellaneous	201

Gas Module:	# of failures
Gas calibration errors	42
Service required errors	17
Plumbing error, sample line blocked	9
Miscellaneous	42

Table 6.1: Tracking equipment failures

The Supplies Component of MESS

Having high quality supplies consistently stocked in their correct location is a challenge in many healthcare settings. Supplies that are out of date or not restocked, or supplies in the wrong location, can dramatically affect a caregiver's ability to maintain a work sequence *consistently*. Like equipment, we need to know four things about each item: the timing, quality, quantity, and location.

Unlike equipment, many supplies are consumed during a work sequence and need replenishment. Various supply chain systems are available for use in healthcare; the basic requirements are as follows:

- Knowing the status of materials at a glance
- Implementing a daily management standard to maintain consistency

- Using the system as a continuous improvement tool

These requirements should be met at the local level and not be solely dependent on a centralized group (e.g., a materials management team) at a distance from the gemba. An example of a locally owned and operated supply chain is the *kanban* system: the consumption requirements (timing, quality, quantity, and location) are printed on kanban cards that signal for replenishing an item when it is used (Figure 6.7).

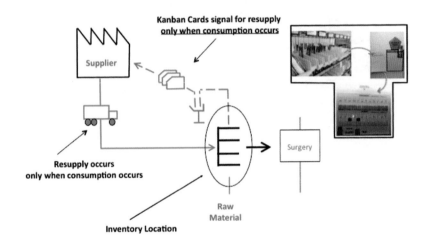

Figure 6.7: Stabilizing the supply system

A typical kanban flow is shown in figure 6.8.

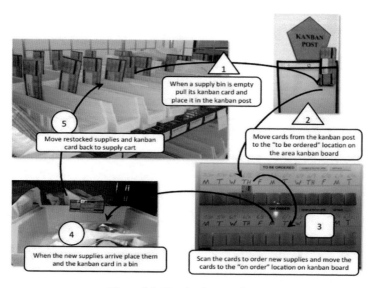

Figure 6.8: How kanban works

Figure 6.8 outlines a lean supply process called kanban, which works in the following way. Step 1, when a supply is depleted, it's kanban card is pulled from the empty bin and moved to a collection point called the kanban post. Several times a day, the cards from the area's kanban posts are moved to the kanban board and placed in the orange row of cardholders that are waiting to be scanned (step 2). In Step 3, the card is scanned, which launches the order for new supplies, and then it is moved into the yellow holder (in this case two days forward, because the lead time for this supply is two days). When new stock arrives, the kanban card is removed from the yellow row where it and the new supplies are placed in the bin (step 4). In step 5, the bin is placed back on the shelf, behind the bin already in use. This is a first-in, first-out (FIFO) system.

Daily management of the kanban process is critical, because kanban is as much a problem-identification tool as a supply-ordering tool. As cards flow through the ordering process, they wind up on a kanban board that is reviewed several times a day. If suppliers deliver supplies late, the area uses more supplies than expected, or if for any other reason the supply system is not functioning as planned, the cards on the board tell the story at a glance. This allows management to see the problem immediately so that it can be fixed and prevented.

The images below (Figure 6.9a,b) show leader standardized work that the person in charge of the kanban system (the kanban coordinator) follows each day to make sure that the supply system is functioning as planned.

Start-of-shift audit (kanban coordinator)

Audit Supply Room: Cycle time = 30 minutes
- Verify that all bins are in compliance with the standard (Bins have items and kanban cards or bins are empty; empty bins have been rotated to the back)
- Verify that there are no supply shortages (at least one full bin is on the cart for every supply, if this is not the case escalate immediately to the manager)
- Take all kanban cards from the post and transfer them to the kanban board
- Write down all supplies issues on the kanban board
- Huddle with charge nurse on supplies status at kanban board

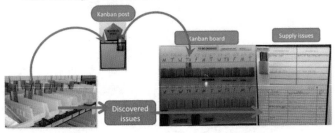

Figure 6.9a: Start of shift management of kanban system

End-of-shift audit (Kanban coordinator)

Audit Supply Room : Cycle time = 30 minutes
- Verify that all bins are in compliance with the standard (Bins have items and kanban cards or bins are empty; empty bins have been rotated to the back)
- Verify that there are no supply shortages (at least 1 full bin is on the cart for every supply, if this is not the case escalate immediately to the manager)
- Take all kanban cards from the post and transfer them to the kanban board
- Record all supply issues on the kanban board
- Huddle with next shift kanban coordinator

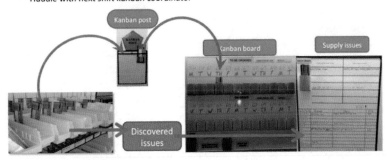

Figure 6.9b: End of shift management of kanban system

The Staff Component of MESS

Stable staffing is necessary for a lean system to function. If an area is short staffed, the people cannot follow a consistent work sequence. Staff may not be available for many reasons: people arrive late or do not show up to work at all, people may be on hand but are not trained for certain procedures, or a staffing plan does not match patient demand.

To resolve the issues that cause unstable staffing, we need to know the next day's patient demand, build a staffing plan that matches that demand, have staff that can flex into multiple roles (via cross-training), and monitor performance through daily management.

Having accurate information to predict what the patient demand will be for the next day can be difficult. After all, patients' conditions change, they can come in late or fail to arrive, providers may have unexpected schedule changes, and emergency admissions can surge. These types of variables can make it difficult to know what might happen tomorrow. How can you get started on stable staffing? Estimate tomorrow's patient demand on an hourly basis, visually post it, and use the data to plan the next day's staffing (Figure 6.10).

Hour	Patients	Doctors required	Nurses required	Medical Assistants required	Clerks Required
8:00	2				
9:00	5				
10:00	5				
11:00	7				
12:00	2				
13:00	5				
14:00	1				
15:00	4				
16:00	1				
17:00	1				

Figure 6.10: Next day's schedule (Demand)

The staffing plan requires understanding how many patients each staff member can handle and then bringing in just enough staff members to cover for the estimated patient demand and necessary breaks. Let's assume that physicians on a unit have a capacity of three patients per hour, nurses have a capacity of four patients, medical assistants have a capacity of seven patients, and clerks have a capacity of six patients. Understanding each member's capacity is critical and depends on thoroughly understanding each member's work sequence (methods) so that staffing levels can be set appropriately.

Table 6.2 shows an example of a daily staffing plan (not including breaks and lunch):

Hour	Patients	Doctors Required	Nurses required	Medical Assistants required	Clerks Required
8:00	2	1	1	1	1
9:00	5	2	2	1	1
10:00	5	2	2	1	1
11:00	7	3	2	1	2
12:00	2	1	1	1	1
13:00	5	2	2	1	1
14:00	1	1	1	1	1
15:00	4	2	1	1	1
16:00	1	1	1	1	1
17:00	1	1	1	1	1

Table 6.2: Next day's schedule & staffing (Demand & Capacity)

Management needs to not only create staffing plans but to also ensure that the staff is flexible enough to respond and do the necessary work. If staff members have only one skill or are allowed to work in only one area, it will be hard to fully use them throughout the day. The solution is to cross-train so they can do different jobs. Ideally, each area team member should be trained in three different work locations, and each work location should have three people trained to do it. This is commonly called the "3 x 3 cross-training goal." A sample cross-training matrix follows (Figure 6.11):

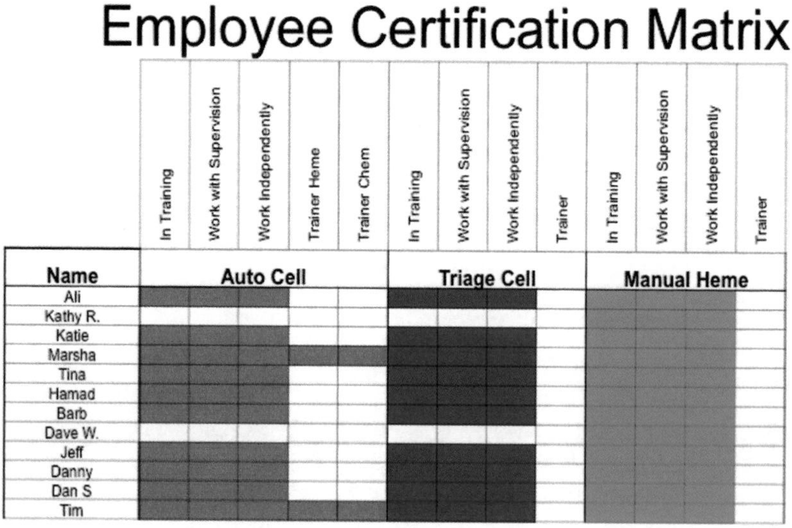

Employee Certification Matrix

Name	Auto Cell					Triage Cell				Manual Heme			
	In Training	Work with Supervision	Work Independently	Trainer Heme	Trainer Chem	In Training	Work with Supervision	Work Independently	Trainer	In Training	Work with Supervision	Work Independently	Trainer
Ali													
Kathy R.													
Katie													
Marsha													
Tina													
Hamad													
Barb													
Dave W.													
Jeff													
Danny													
Dan S													
Tim													

Figure 6.11: Employee cross training matrix

In addition to creating flexibility in an area, cross-training can lead to sharing resources across units, which provides even more opportunity to provide consistent work for staff while maximizing operational efficiency. A shared nursing pool is an example of taking this idea to its furthest extent.

5S

A common place to start lean is workplace organization or 5S (Figure 6.12). Just like a messy garage is difficult to work in, a disorganized workplace wastes caregivers' time while they search for the items they need. The 5S process is a time-tested, visually oriented system that creates and maintains greater organization, efficiency, and safety while reducing training time, search time, and wasted time and resources. Each S stands for an organizational activity: sort (separate as needed), simplify (create a place for everything), sweep (create a visual workplace), standardize (document), and sustain (hold the gains through leader standardized work).

5S for Workplace Organization

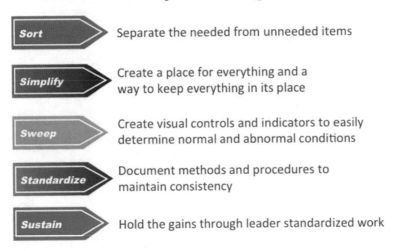

Sort — Separate the needed from unneeded items

Simplify — Create a place for everything and a way to keep everything in its place

Sweep — Create visual controls and indicators to easily determine normal and abnormal conditions

Standardize — Document methods and procedures to maintain consistency

Sustain — Hold the gains through leader standardized work

Figure 6.12: 5S definition

The 5S improvement events can get frontline workers engaged in lean transformations, because their work becomes easier. A side benefit of 5S is improved compliance with regulatory standards such as ensuring egress (hallways and rooms are properly cleared of equipment).

Level 2 Culture

Although lean methods typically get most of the attention and energy, level 2 is at least as much about cultural change as it is about the tools. A simple definition of culture is "what the workforce does when management is not watching." When lean transformations fail, it is often because the culture and attitudes haven't changed rather than because the lean tools or methods don't work. That's why it is important to also focus on the cultural transformation. An excellent resource, listed in the bibliography, for studying lean culture can be found in David Mann's book entitled, *"Creating a Lean Culture: Tools to Sustain Lean Conversions."*

Clinician and Staff Development

This is the first time that most clinicians and staff will have the opportunity to experience and learn about lean processes. Level 2 improvements can build enthusiasm because they tend to make the staff's work easier. Better availability of the things needed to do the job efficiently, thanks to MESS, is rarely seen as a bad thing. The only downside is difficulty maintaining the gains. As with all lean transformations, greater efficiency is obtained by implementing greater daily operational rigor. Getting used to the increased rigor of consistently maintaining work sequences at all levels will take time and help from management.

Physician Engagement

Engaging physicians in the lean improvement work is essential. Without their involvement, countermeasures for care processes will miss an important voice, and the result will be partial solutions. Relatively short, focused lean education sessions should be tailored to the physician. Ideally, this education would be followed by participation in an improvement event. As Jack Billi claims, "Lean is practical to its core. Helping physicians to 'learn it by doing it' can help overcome resistance. When physicians can see for themselves that scientific problem solving improves patients' experience and at the same time makes it easier for them to do their work, most become converts. For this reason, I suggest always scoping a problem or project to ensure it includes some of the physician's pain with the current process."

As lean organizations mature, they often form kaizen operations teams or LITs. These teams require ongoing physician input to help them solve difficult issues. It is important to accept that this work cannot be an unfunded mandate for physicians. The organization must remunerate the physicians for their time in improvement events and as members of an LIT. For physicians in leadership roles who receive medical direction funds from their healthcare systems, a portion of the funds should go to support the time needed to improve both clinical and nonclinical processes. Clinical standardized work (care pathways) is a good example of worthy processes to be defined and improved with deep physician involvement and leadership. This requires an exhaustive review of the literature, a deep understanding of the organization's patient population, and a robust analytics department.

Activate Everyone

In a successful lean transformation, everyone must become involved, because lean can work only as a team effort. Everyone should dance to the same tune as quickly as possible so that the results can be maximized as soon as possible. Types of unengaged groups and countermeasures for them include the following:

- *Preoccupied people who don't want to spend time on a lean transformation, although they are typically fine with others who want to try it.* The countermeasure is education. Start by explaining the improvements that lean will deliver to the customer but include staff and business concerns. With that knowledge, it's easier to bring preoccupied team members aboard.
- *Those with no opportunity to be involved, which is common among frontline staff.* The countermeasure is to have management create a plan to increase the opportunity to participate. This can be done via rapid process improvement workshops, training sessions, or daily staffled improvements, coupled with staffing plans that allow time for improvement work.
- *Those who feel scared to engage in the lean transformation.* Everyone needs to feel safe to experiment and fail at improving processes. Until managers act as true lean leaders, this will not be possible. Failure should be embraced as an opportunity for improvement, not as anyone's fault. Some fear that the lean efforts will result in a loss of jobs due to enhanced productivity and the need for fewer people. This should not occur—it will kill a lean transformation.
- *Those who are uninterested in changing.* Although typically a minority, this group will need to be addressed as soon as possible if the transformation is to succeed. Education, coupled with coaching from lean leaders, is needed. For this group, it's common to hide from

doing lean work, hoping that it will pass. The good news is that as the executive and management teams start to become lean leaders, their frequency in the gemba greatly increases, and people are not allowed to hide. Publicly celebrating success will also increase awareness and understanding for this group.

Management Development

The frontline worker's primary job is to follow and improve standardized work. It is the primary job of management (including senior management and executives) to help the frontline workers achieve and improve their standardized work.

In level 2, managers (from frontline to executives) need to make the time to be in their areas much more than a traditional system required. Lean systems are built to surface problems, and if management is not there to help with the issues that arise, the improvements will quickly revert to the original state. Once the managers' time is sufficiently freed, structured daily reviews of their areas from the end of the patients' flow to the beginning should be introduced. This daily review, commonly called a "gemba round," should be done with the entire management team. The idea of gemba rounds is threefold:

- To make the management team knowledgeable on issues throughout the unit so they can help solve problems
- To give a daily cadence for the team to ask for help with the problems that impede workflow
- To tie the unit's issues into one group so that they can be prioritized and solved in their order of importance to overall unit flow (this is a way to break down siloed thinking)

To quickly facilitate this review, each subarea (if there are subareas) displays a management board, which the management group visits during the gemba round. In figure 6.13, the team is huddled around boards posted on the outside of an OR. The team is reviewing the day's turnover times and case length times (scheduled versus actual) for that room.

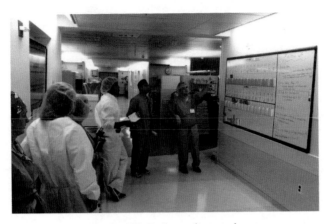

Figure 6.13: Daily gemba rounds

Role of a Level 2 Lean Leader

The following examples illustrate the role of a level 2 lean leader.

Scenario 1: Betty is a nurse manager who is struggling to sustain 5S in her area. She feels overwhelmed with her workload and now has to deal with a 5S initiative that she did not ask for. An experienced lean manager would understand that it is unfair to think that Betty can solve this issue by herself. Betty should expect help from her manager to determine what is most important—her current work or the 5S initiative—or to determine what needs to be reprioritized or dropped so that she can attend the 5S initiative. Typically, schedules include extraneous work (such as meetings) that will need to be reprioritized so that lean transformation work can be done.

Scenario 2: Dr. Dodge, a surgeon, has been asked to participate in some lean events to improve OR turnover time. She replies that she cannot, because her schedule won't allow her to attend. An experienced lean manager would talk privately, communicating to her the importance of the work and to understand why Dr. Dodge can't be available. If Dr. Dodge still cannot participate, a substitute surgeon should be chosen. If no surgeons can attend, the issue needs to be

141

escalated to the executive team immediately so that it can remove barriers and garner the much-needed surgeon input. Lean leadership at the executive level requires that executives rectify these situations immediately so that transformation work can proceed.

A lean leader helps solve the issues that area workers cannot on their own so that the frontline team can continue its work. In both scenarios, if Betty and Dr. Dodge were not supported by a lean leader, the lean work would have stopped or proceeded in a suboptimal fashion.

Another hallmark of a lean leader is the ability to inspire people to take action and solve problems at the lowest possible level. A lean leader must gather data the old-fashioned way using The Three Actuals rule. As issues are spotted, it is critical not to jump too quickly to solutions. Almost every problem can be tied to a management failing, so before you ask, "How could this happen?" ask, "How can I help?" Leaders (including executives) should go to the gemba as frequently as possible, certainly no less than weekly, and do nothing more than observe processes. Ask oneself, "Is it obvious if we are on track or not?" If it's not obvious to the leader observing at the gemba, chances are that it's not obvious to those working in the area. In this case, a lean leader would work with the area staff and leaders to formulate plans for the necessary improvements.

Daily Management Consists of Two Parts

Daily management is built in two sections. One is supporting the frontline workers by responding to abnormalities. The other is supporting corporate strategic goals. This two-pronged management approach requires each level of management to be aware of what the levels above and below them require (Figure 6.14).

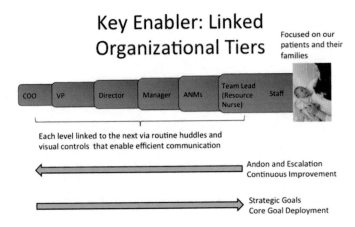

Figure 6.14: Linkage of organizational tiers

Figure 6.15 breaks down the duties of each management level to support both operational and strategic goals.

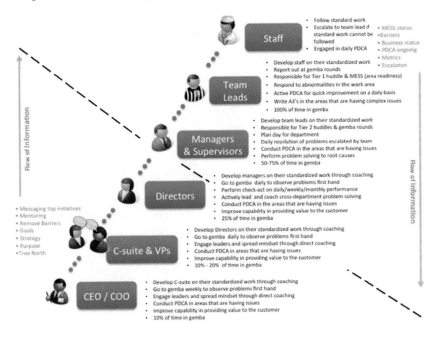

Figure 6.15: Daily management duties (*See page 245 for expanded view of figure 6.15)

The importance of all levels of management doing supportive work in the gemba every day cannot be overstated. Perhaps the single biggest mistake managers can make is to think that the gemba time will be in addition to the "regular work." The paradigm needs to change to the statement, "This *is* the work." To do this, leaders should book this time into their daily schedules and create detailed, leader standardized work that outlines work sequences during these times. Each level of leadership should reinforce the daily leader standardized work of the levels below. This creates a nested structure that keeps the system working at all levels. By nature, standards at all levels are in a continuous state of decline, and leader standardized work keeps the unit operating at maximum potential (Figure 6.16a–c).

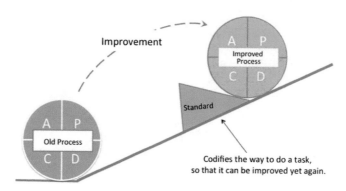

Figure 6.16a: Standards hold process improvement gains

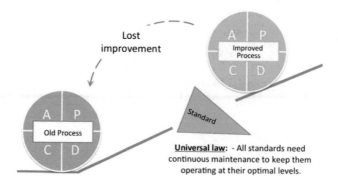

Figure 6.16b: Standards erode over time

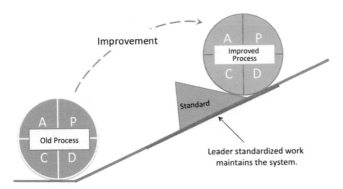

Figure 6.16c: Leader standardized work: Holds process improvement
gains by maintaining the standards

Leader Standardized Work

Leader standardized work should include start-of-shift, end-of-shift, and mid-shift components (Figure 6.17). At the start of a shift, it is critical to verify area readiness. This is done by verifying that MESS components are all in place and ready for the day's demand. The end-of-shift portion should aim at verifying that a good handoff to the next shift will be made. This is primarily done by verifying that MESS components are all in place before the first shift leaves. Auditing the areas in real time as the day progresses is last.

Layout for Leader Standardized Work

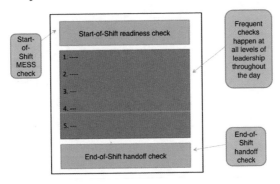

Figure 6.17: Layout for leader standardized work by shift

As previously stated, leader standardized work is structured so that one level of leadership checks the level below (Figure 6.18). Variation at any level is identified and continuously improved.

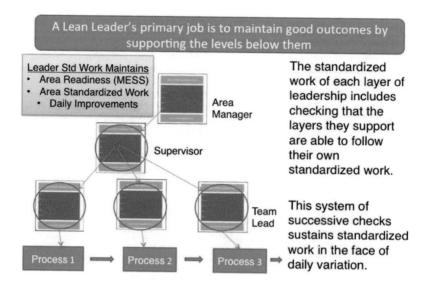

Figure 6.18: Leader standardized work

Quick Hits and Big Issues

A final component is a system that collects the issues (problems) discovered during the day's auditing (Table 6.3). Issues typically break down into two categories. Quick hits are issues that are easy to take care of in a relatively short time (usually twenty-four to forty-eight hours) and are usually completed within the affected work unit.

Gemba Walk's Quick Hit List

Date	Location	Owner	Issue	Action	Resolve Date	Completed?
22-Aug	SSU	Bev	Patients arriving at appt time, not early enough for admitting	appt with Diane Flynn to write letter to parents	23-Aug	
22-Aug	SSU	Bev	Who's job is it to ensure pts arrive on time?	Bev to pull andon, email Denise unifying units/policy to keep pts on time	25-Aug	
22-Aug	APU	Bev	green!			
22-Aug	PAC U	Wendy	Post-op note quick solutions are skewing the overall data	Pause collection of post-op note data, add transportation onto the PACU audits	24-Aug	
22-Aug	Materials	Nancy	Kanbans red	Nancy to make announcement about Kanban carts	23-Aug	
22-Aug	SPD	Linda	Kanbans	Work in Progress!	23-Aug	
22-Aug	OR	Nancy	OR whiteboards unorganized and difficult to read	Reorganize--SPD, OR, Materials	23-Aug	
22-Aug	Scheduling	Emily	Cardiac scheduling patients within frozen period	Decipher how to track Cardiac pts	23-Aug	
22-Aug	PAC	May Jung	no quick hits			

Through Gemba rounds, managers are able to see and resolve minor issues every day!

Table 6.3: Quick hits

The second set of problems to be solved, "big issues," will take days, weeks, or months to fix, often due to their complexity or multidisciplinary nature. An example of a big issues board follows below (Figure 6.19). The board needs to include the following:

1. The date the issue was observed
2. A description of the issue
3. The owner of the issue (typically an area manager)
4. A major milestone that can be addressed quickly (within one week)
5. A target date for milestone completion
6. Whether it is on track (in green) or not (in red)

Only one big issue per owner can be on the board so it can be worked on and eliminated as soon as possible. Once a big issue is solved, it is removed, and the owner can take on another.

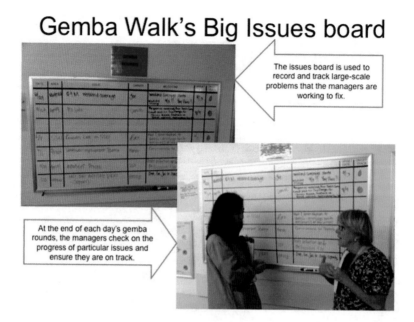

Figure 6.19: Big issues board

Executives' Role in Level 2

Engaging and supporting the frontline staff is important, but so is learning how to be an engaged executive. Because acquiring basic stability depends largely on engaging frontline staff through successful improvement events, executives at this stage often applaud the frontline but limit their own roles to being spectators of the improved "hockey game." Better hockey needs to be practiced *with* executives; otherwise, the advancement of lean throughout the organization tends to stall. Disengaged executive teams ask others to explain the return on investment for lean, why the organization is not going fast enough, or why metrics met at prior improvement events are slipping. They need to be deeply attached to the transformation work and answering such questions by seeing with their own eyes.

Posting an executive scorecard in the executive conference room can be helpful. Such scorecard should monitor things like weekly presence in the gemba, huddle attendance in the gemba, the number of A3s or improvement events each executive has sponsored per month, attendance at all-hands improvement report-out events, and gemba time booked and being followed. Together, these practices are deemed leader (executive) standardized work for the day or the week. They should be collated into a leader standardized work calendar and their completion tracked.

Engagement by Doing

Senior managers and executives with and without clinical backgrounds will need to start their own personal lean transformations by going to the gemba frequently (at least once per week) and diving deeply into the defects by engaging frontline workers and their managers in problem solving. This requires personally getting into the details and spending the necessary time to help solve the problems. Until senior managers understand that this will be their new primary role, a high-functioning lean system will not be possible.

Key points regarding executives and gemba engagement include the following:

1. Executives, and all managers, need to pick the right problems to work on. They should not confuse the organization by attacking every problem they see. Executives should pick critical issues (no more than one or two at the start) and be relentless in helping to solve these issues. If areas are having difficulty solving the critical issues at their root, it is incumbent upon the executive team to do whatever is necessary to solve the issue.

   To start, go see the following conditions. Where what is observed does not meet the standard, help to correct the process:

   a. Is 5S meeting expectations?
   b. Is patient experience meeting expectations (care area that is warm, quiet, well lit, uncluttered, with empathetic staff)?
   c. Do safety and quality measures meet expectations?
   d. Are teamwork and problem-solving capabilities meeting expectations?

2. This work can be done only in the gemba, not from a conference room or office. Executives should not demand change from those in the gemba without following up themselves. Their absence from the gemba is often viewed as a lack of true commitment, especially early in a lean journey, when the organization is wondering if the executive team is serious about the new management system or if it will wither with time.

3. Executives should not work *around* area management when helping solve problems. They should work *with* area management to solve key issues quickly. When deviations to the standard are observed, the natural response of executives is to solve the problem quickly using the best way they know how. This is how many senior managers ascended in their careers: immediate problem solving and knowing the answers. However, the first step should be to get area managers involved immediately to solve the problem with the manager's team. Where area managers say they are encountering barriers to successful or expeditious countermeasures, the executives' role is to provide the resources or facilitation needed.

4. Lean executives need to be relentless. Problems are always harder to solve at their root than they think they will be. That's why the critical issues that *must* be solved are the ones to start with. Once executives understand how tough this is, they will be more humble in the future. They will have been communicating to the staff that they are serious about solving the frontline's critical issues and that the organization is committed to using lean to solve those issues. This will give the frontline improvements a huge boost. Follow-up is critical to show support for the process, to celebrate results, and to see if the intended outcomes were consistently reached. If consistency is an issue, executives need to go back to the drawing board with area managers and staff and support a new set of countermeasures. (Expect a lot of this.) This is nothing more than the PDCA cycle.

We suggest that senior managers start their own transformations by picking one persistent quality defect that clearly needs to be solved for reasons of patient safety.

Although there are many candidates, we suggest something that is fundamentally important, widespread, and easy to understand such as proper hand hygiene. Senior managers should go to the gemba and ask for data on the area's hand hygiene compliance. If there are no data, they should sponsor (and be part of) a lean event with the team to build the standards and measures that the area will follow regarding this critical process. Once agreement is reached and the new standards are launched, the work is only beginning, because there is bound to be backsliding. Senior managers need to follow up every time they visit the gemba with the following actions:

1. Ask the manager, "How is your hand hygiene performance against the standard?"
2. Stand in the area for an extended period (at least thirty minutes), and observe the actual people performing the actual task. Compare the observations with the data reported in step 1.
3. Where variances are witnessed, talk to the team members who deviated from the standard (not their manager), and in a respectful manner, learn why the standard was not followed. Do not criticize, and do not act on the first data point.
4. Talk to other frontline team members to gain further information and deepen understanding about why the defect is occurring.
5. Once deep understanding of the problem is achieved, act to help solve the issue.
   a. If the frontline reported that no hand sanitizer was available, the senior manager can coach the area manager to partner with housekeeping and set a new standard for hand sanitizer availability. Employ this new standard quickly!
   b. If the frontline staff reports that they did not know about the standard, the senior manager and area manager can review a training plan and any gaps or barriers. Employ this new standard quickly!
   c. If the frontline staff reports that the standard is confusing and hard to follow, the senior manager can confer with the

area manager and staff and help to make the standard easier to understand and follow. Employ this new standard quickly!

6. As senior managers become facile with this activity, their actions encourage junior managers to act with the same focus and speed, which will greatly speed up problem solving in the gemba.

Seeing for yourself in the workplace and acting on findings is a never-ending cycle, because there will always be defects to be addressed. This approach is hands on and different from the traditional "cheerleading" approach, but it is necessary for transformation.

Once executives become proficient with their standardized work, including problem solving deep dives, they must continue to sharpen their lean skills by becoming lean mentors. They can learn about the work in a deep way by observing the areas in action. They should pick an important problem and work with area leaders to solve the issue. This is as much about building engaged leaders and staff as it is about problem solving. Executives must do A3s on the issues that they see that are impeding frontline workers. Great leaders and staff are the product of great executives.

For more information on this, we suggest that executives and lean practitioners read *The Toyota Mindset: The Ten Commandments of Taiichi Ohno,*[19] which outlines this approach in detail. It does a nice job of explaining how Ohno acted as a senior executive at Toyota, with many examples of him standing in the gemba and facilitating problem solving based on what he observed.

Level 2 Mindset

The mindset change at this level is that lean is learned by doing. No amount of classroom training can develop the problem solving capabilities, team support, management behaviors, and esprit dé corps necessary to create operational stability. Mindsets need to change from collating, storing, and managing information on a clipboard, to making the basic requirements for area readiness (MESS) visible. The lean team comes together to share information about area readiness, quickly solve issues getting in the way of the patient's safe journey, and escalate big issues that require a senior manager's help or cross-functional input.

This lean level mandates that all managers understand that they need to start managing downward; that is, supporting the front line. This is difficult and will take time, because much of present-day management is managing up—making the boss(es) happy. Lean management is about supporting the frontline workers, whose focus is to make patients happy, which is the ultimate goal—thus the bosses will be happy too.

CHAPTER 7

Level 3—Matching
Capacity to Demand

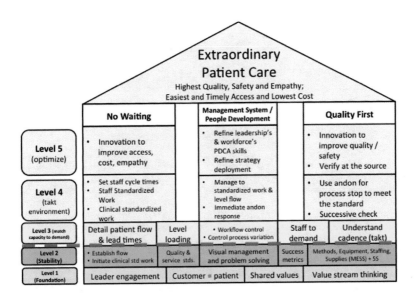

Achieving operational stability in level 2 sets the stage for consistent performance each time a clinical worker executes a task. In level 3, we create the tempo of an advanced lean healthcare system by calculating the cadence (takt time) of patient demand and aligning staff and clinician work around that patient flow. Our graphic of the lean house has a dotted red line, between levels 2 and 3 which, as previously described in Chapter 4, depicts the beginning of an *advanced* lean transformation. This is where patient flow times are calculated. The other principle of level 3 work, matching staff capacity to patient demand, will necessitate significant changes in scheduling processes.

Slow and Steady Wins the Race

As in Aesop's fable of the hare and the tortoise, a slow and steady work pace wins the race. Workflow is much more efficient when it runs like consistent tortoises (ballet) rather than sporadic hares (hockey). Unfortunately, slow and steady is not the traditional healthcare model—sometimes for good reason but often not.

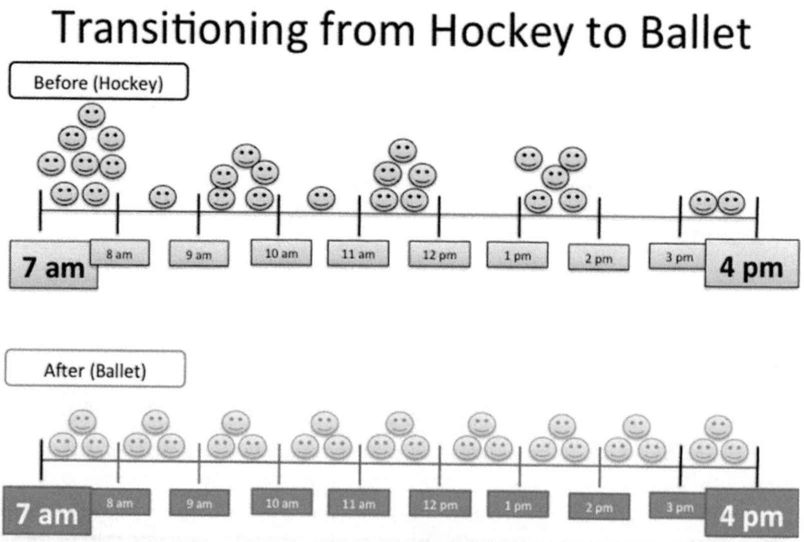

Figure 7.1: Traditional vs. lean flow

The goal of a leveled operation is to exactly match capacity (the number of staff and clinicians) to demand (the number of patients). To get started, we need to understand what drives nonlevel flow of daily operations in healthcare.

Hourly capacity and demand are variable in the traditional healthcare setting because of the following:

a. Patients are not scheduled in a level fashion, so they arrive in large boluses. As shown in figure 7.1 above, at various times (7:00, 9:00, 11:00, and 1:00), the staff is overburdened due to high patient volume, and at other times (8:00 and 10:00 am and 12:00, 2:00, and 3:00 pm), they have very little patient work.

b. In the OR setting, some surgeons don't want to perform surgeries on Fridays or later than 3:00 p.m. This drives hospitals to build and staff ORs that would not be needed in a leveled system.

c. Staffing shift lengths are not matched to demand. For example, staff in a recovery room work twelve-hour shifts, but the demand is for a shorter shift, so the organization pays direct labor costs for unused capacity.

d. Patients have urgent needs that can't wait for a scheduled time. There will always be a need for urgent care. The key is to view this part of the business as just that—*part* of the business but not the *whole* business—and devise systems that take this variable into account.

e. Staffing plans do not account for absenteeism, so those who do show up get overwhelmed.

Linking Capacity to Demand Matching and Quality

Imagine that you are a nurse on an inpatient unit who knows that properly admitting a new patient from the recovery room takes fifteen minutes. The key steps are to obtain a high quality handoff from the recovery room nurse, verify the physician's orders, make sure the patient's equipment is operating correctly, and input the necessary entries into the EHR. Now imagine that a large volume of patients, all of whom need to be admitted at once, force the nurse to spend only five minutes on each admission. What critical steps might she cut to get to the next patient? What if she doesn't skip steps but does everything at breakneck speed? What are the chances of an adverse quality event under these conditions?

Without capacity consistently matched to demand, clinical staff members frequently face these kinds of hard decisions. This is why the first step of healthcare ballet is to define the cadence (takt time) at which patients need to be served. Once we know the cadence, it is relatively simple to match capacity with demand so that workers aren't overburdened, forced to cut corners, or at risk for quality issues. For the inpatient nurse, as long as the patient flow never exceeds her capacity of one admission every fifteen minutes, all the steps necessary for a high quality admission will be possible.

If we stop and think about how widespread nonleveled flow is throughout healthcare and consider its adverse effects on care quality—such as medication errors when nurses are overwhelmed by patient care duties due to inadequate staffing—it is obvious that capacity must match demand.

Aligning around Patient Flow (The Value Stream)

Hockey is time based. When the game clock reads zero, the scores are tallied, a winner is announced, and someone loses. By contrast, ballet is destination based. The goal is to smoothly thread a storyline together from a known starting point to a predetermined end, at which point everyone is satisfied. Building a destination-based approach in healthcare is important, and to do that, we need to build our storyline around the patient's journey through the system from beginning to end.

Although the value stream approach was discussed in earlier chapters, its adoption becomes critical in the areas undergoing advanced lean transformation. Without smooth patient flow from start to finish (a storyline) that everyone understands and is working to support, areas working on process improvement will not be able to get past level 2 (better hockey).

Figure 7.2 is a value stream view of a patient who requires a surgical procedure. If we attempt to level capacity to demand by creating a level flow through one area in the journey without leveling flow in the other areas, the ballet we are trying to create will quickly be destroyed. For example, if the preoperative (preop) area has a level patient flow but the ORs do not, the OR's inability to flow will quickly back up the patients in preop, destroying any chance of a level patient flow there.

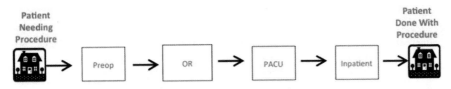

Figure 7.2: Perioperative services value stream

Similarly, if the OR can level patient flow but the post-anesthesia care unit (PACU) or recovery room cannot, the PACU's inability to support patient flow stops patients from exiting ORs, which destroys any chance of level flow in the ORs. We must look at all the interconnected points of the patient's journey as *one flow* instead of making one particular area more efficient.

When aligning by a value stream, it is crucial to start at the exit point of the patient flow you wish to optimize and work backward since the exit point acts as the pacemaker for the patient's journey.

Setting a Pacemaker to Pull the Work through the Value Stream

It is helpful to think of each station or care unit in the value stream as a link in a chain. The stations are loosely connected and maintain a straight line as long as they are pulled from the end of the value stream. If they're pushed from behind, they bunch up. Patient flow should look like a straight line rather than one that is being pushed (Figure 7.3).

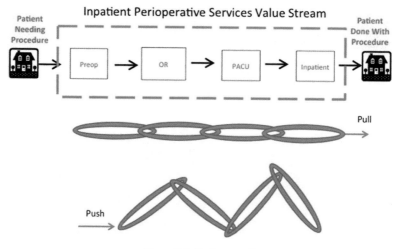

Figure 7.3: Push vs. pull

A push from behind would be analogous to the preop team, at its discretion, sending patients forward in the care journey. The OR, PACU, or inpatient units, based on space or staff capacity, would be unable to serve them. As many of us know, this is an everyday reality in healthcare. When the PACU is ready to transfer or push a patient to an inpatient unit, the inpatient unit is often not ready, and the patient care chain gets bunched up. Patients stay in the PACU too long, occupying beds that could be used by those finishing their surgical procedures. The whole value stream backs up, and patients and clinicians end up waiting.

The key is to pull the end of a chain. The last station needs to be set as the pacemaker that *pulls* the work through the chain and matches capacity with demand (Figure 7.4).

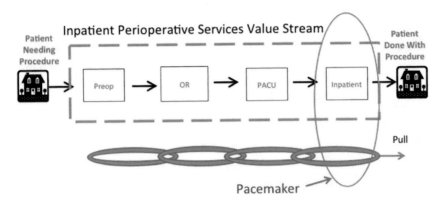

Figure 7.4: Setting the pacemaker

With the value stream defined by the flow created by a pull at the end, the next task is to incorporate patient demand (takt time) and work process times (cycle times) in order to maintain level flow.

Calculating the Cadence (Takt Time)

Now that we have a value stream defining our storyline, we need to come up with the tempo of our ballet. In healthcare, the cadence of any process needs to be the pace at which patients come in the doors. Otherwise, patients will be sitting in waiting rooms or staff will be waiting for the next patient to appear. The cadence of patient demand in a value stream is called "takt time." This is the rate at which the system needs to serve patients. It is a calculation based on the minutes available to work divided by the number of patients demanding to be served in that time.

For example, what takt time (minutes per patient) should we design the system in figure 7.5 to handle?

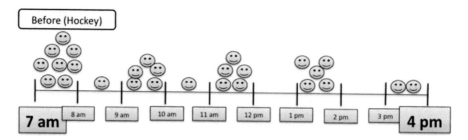

Figure 7.5: Before level flow

Simple math reveals that over the first four hours, the following occurs:

- In the first hour, the rate is 8 patients per hour or 7.5 minutes per patient.
- In the second hour, the rate is 1 patient per hour or 60 minutes per patient.
- In the third hour, the rate is 5 patients per hour or 12 minutes per patient.
- In the fourth hour, the rate is 1 patient per hour or 60 minutes per patient.

This work quantity per hour is highly variable, which drives the available time for each patient's care from 7.5 minutes to more than sixty minutes, depending on the hour of the day.

If we go back to the inpatient admission nurse who needed fifteen minutes to perform a high-quality admission from the recovery room, in the hours with four or fewer patients to be admitted, one nurse could perform the process without risking an adverse quality event. Said another way, if only one nurse is available, overburden is more likely to cause quality errors during the hours of 7:00, 9:00, 11:00, and 1:00. One way of solving the overburden issue would be to flex nurses in and out to match capacity with demand. If a nurse needs fifteen minutes to do the job, the number of nurses required per hour, and hence their utilization (productivity), is calculated in table 7.1 using the patient data from figure 7.5.

Time	Number of nurses	Utilization
7:00 a.m.	2	100 percent
8:00 a.m.	1	25 percent
9:00 a.m.	2	63 percent
10:00a.m.	1	25 percent
11:00 a.m.	2	63 percent

Table 7.1: Productivity Data

In theory, matching capacity with demand can be done with flexible staffing, but as suggested by the example, it is nearly impossible to move staff enough to match highly variable demand patterns. The preferred way to level the workload is to level demand so that staffing remains constant.

Consider the same number of patients served in the same time but with level demand, as shown in the figure 7.6:

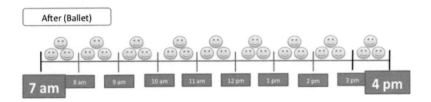

Figure 7.6: After level flow

Using the ideal leveled system in figure 7.6, what takt time should we design our system to handle? Math reveals the following:

- In the first hour, the rate is 3 patients per hour or 20 minutes per patient.
- In the second hour, the rate is 3 patient per hour or 20 minutes per patient.
- In the third hour, the rate is 3 patients per hour or 20 minutes per patient.

- In the fourth hour, the rate is 3 patient per hour or 20 minutes per patient.

The leveled workflow has a consistent rate of three patients per hour (one every twenty minutes). Notice that with this level patient flow, the takt time is unchanging. This is the easiest flow to staff against.

Using our example, we would calculate takt time as follows:

The total time available = 9 hours (7:00 a.m. to 4:00 p.m.) = 540 minutes
The total number of patients served = 27
The takt time = 540/27 = 20 minutes/patient

Because the takt time is the rate at which the value stream needs to serve its patients, it is important to first define the patient group you want to build an advanced lean system around. Map the areas they visit during their stays (the beginning and end of that value stream), and draw a box around those areas. Two sample value streams are outlined below (Figure 7.7a,b) that so their takt times can be calculated.

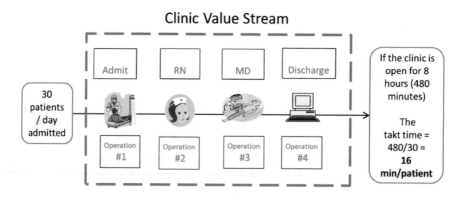

Figure 7.7a: Clinic value stream

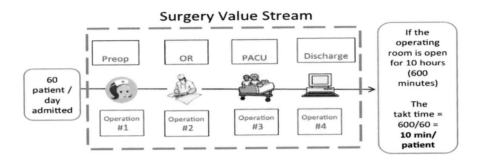

Figure 7.7b: Surgery value stream

Once the box has been drawn around the areas involved in the patient's flow through the value stream, use the number of patients entering and leaving that boxed area as the denominator and the total daily hours available to serve them as the numerator.

Leveling Demand in ORs

Although different areas will require their own specific leveling systems, the basics are always the same: understand the historical patient demand, calculate the takt time, and schedule one patient per takt time. Building on our previous example, these steps are illustrated in Figures 7.8a–d for leveling capacity to demand in ORs.

Step 1. Understand the historical patient volume (the demand curve).

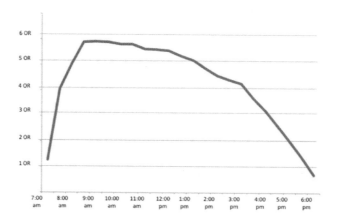

Figure 7.8a: Operating room demand

When the demand curve is not level throughout the day, a new level/demand model will need to be created. In this case, the hospital wanted to support a capacity of thirty surgeries per day and wanted a level loaded ten-hour window in which to perform all thirty procedures, resulting in the demand curve in figure 7.8b.

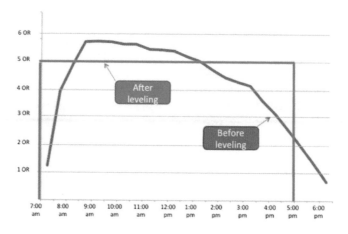

Figure 7.8b: Operating room demand before and after leveling

Step 2. Because the new model will be designed to handle a demand of thirty surgeries in a ten-hour day, the following takt calculation is used (Figure 7.8c).

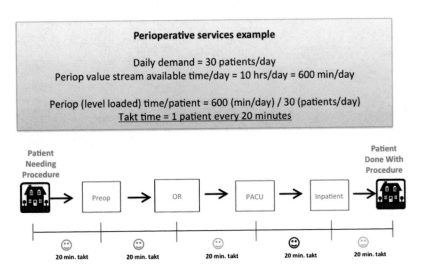

Figure 7.8c: Takt time calculation example

Step 3. Now that the takt time has been calculated, we need to invent a scheduling system that schedules one patient every takt (twenty minutes) as shown in Figure 7.8d.

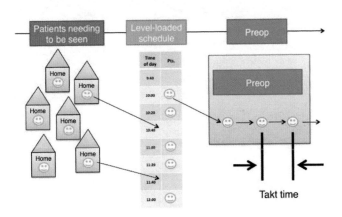

Figure 7.8d: Creating a level schedule

The facility in our example has seven operating rooms with a broad variety of case types and lengths. All the cases are broken into how many takt times (twenty-minute segments) they represent and then arranged so that one case ends every takt period. This ensures that one patient flows into the PACU every twenty minutes, which also means that preop has to supply a new patient to the ORs only every twenty minutes. In this way, staff overburden is reduced and patient care quality is increased.

An example of a theoretical leveled schedule is depicted in figure 7.9. The colored rectangles are different surgical procedures, with their varying lengths representing the allotted time for each procedure. Two days before a scheduled procedure, the cases are arranged so that they end, as much as possible, in twenty-minute increments, thus delivering one patient to the PACU every twenty minutes

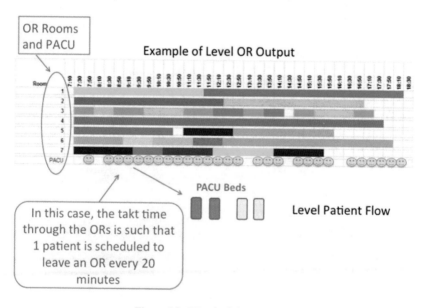

Figure 7.9: OR scheduling system

The picture below (figure 7.10) shows an actual OR level scheduling tool. Inside the rectangles, which denote case length, are notes for each procedure's detail: estimated time, special equipment or additional surgeons needed, etc.

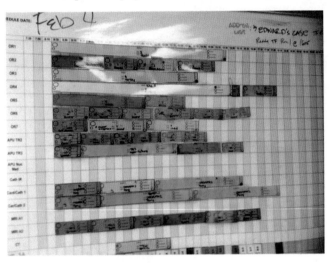

Figure 7.10: Actual OR scheduling board

Step 4. Once the takt time and level scheduling mechanisms are understood, it is time to implement a level scheduling process that stretches from the initial clinic request for surgery to the day of surgery. Figure 7.11 shows how surgical appointments more than fifteen days from the surgery date are maintained at the clinics (not the OR) and are considered in a phase of scheduling known as "liquid"—these appointments can be changed without affecting the OR schedule, which tracks only cases within fifteen days of the procedure. The moment the appointments flow into the OR scheduling system, they are considered "slushy"—firming up but not yet set in stone—at which time insurance authorization is confirmed and special anesthesia considerations are worked up. Cases can still change at this phase, but the effort hospital staff spends on slushy cases is not trivial, so it is important that clinics confirm with patients and physicians that the appointment is correct before it proceeds to OR scheduling. Two days prior to the surgery, the cases are "frozen" into the OR schedule by level loading them into twenty minute takt times using the process described earlier.

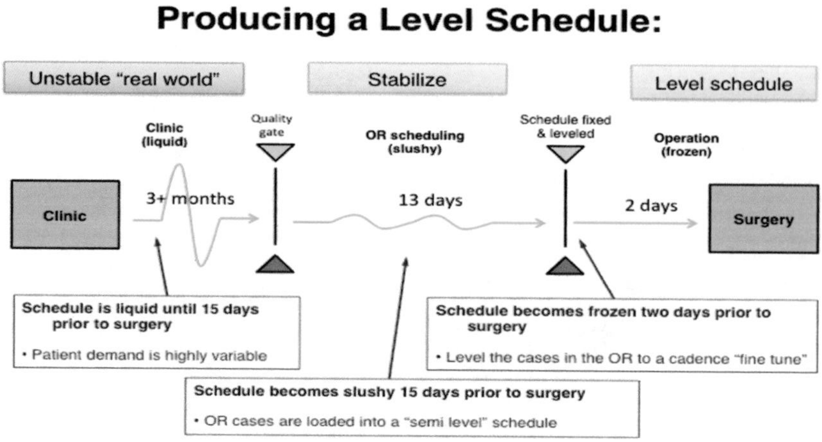

Producing a Level Schedule:

Figure 7.11: Scheduling process

Leveling Demand in Inpatient Units

Like OR leveling, we start by understanding historical patient demand and then calculating the takt time.

Step 1. Inpatient flow varies from day to day, so the historical demand graph should start with a daily view. In figure 7.12 from an actual inpatient unit, notice that the demand averages eleven patients per day but can range from twenty-three to one. How many patients per day should we design the system to serve?

The answer is not as scientific as it is business minded. In all businesses, risk and reward must be measured to set up a system for optimal output. Using the demand data plus near-term market growth potential, the team decided to design the system to twenty discharges per day. Twenty discharges rarely happened in the last year, so for days with fewer than twenty discharges, the system had more capacity than needed. This extra capacity had to be monitored and the system changed if demand didn't increase as predicted.

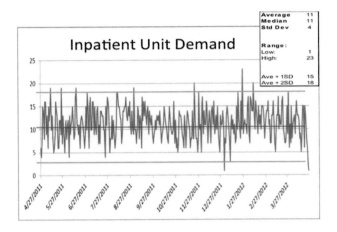

Figure 7.12: Inpatient demand

Inpatient unit flow is as much about getting patients out (discharge) as getting them in (admission). For this reason, we like to superimpose admission and discharge when looking at inpatient units. Figure 7.13a shows a large spike in discharges but no spike in admissions. The discharge spike is driven by two factors. First, patients don't want to leave in the middle of the night, and this factor can't be changed easily, so it must be factored into the discharge hours. Second, hospital discharge policy affects discharge hours, creating this demand spike; the hours being used for discharge are principally 10:00 a.m. to 4:00 p.m. Note that admissions (labeled as input) are relatively level.

Inpatient Average Admissions & Discharges, by Hour

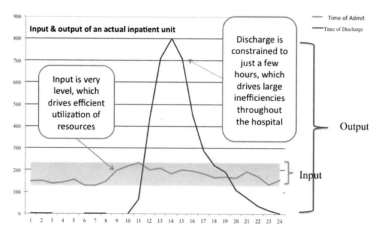

Figure 7.13a: Inpatient admit and discharge data

Step 2. Now that the business has set patient demand at twenty patients per day, we need to level discharges by opening the time window for discharge (Figure 7.13b). In this case, the unit set up new policies and procedures to support discharges from 8:00 a.m. to 6:00 p.m. (ten hours). We can calculate the discharge takt time: 20 patients/10 hours = 2 patients per hour.

Discharges from an Inpatient Unit

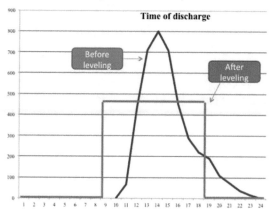

Figure 7.13b: Leveling inpatient discharge

Expanding the discharge hours and leveling patient flow to two patients per hour enables all hospital services for this unit (physicians, nurses, social services, physical therapy, and pharmacy) to work more efficiently. All services benefit by not having to deal with a discharge spike (Figure 7.13c).

Before and after leveling discharge

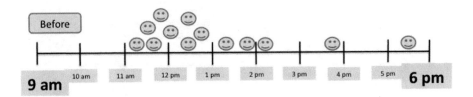

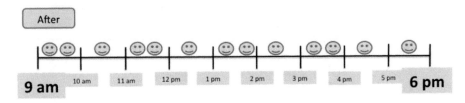

Figure 7.13c: Traditional vs. level Inpatient discharge

Step 3. Like the OR, the inpatient unit needs a mechanism that maintains a level schedule so that patients leave when planned at a takt time of two per hour. This is the function of the discharge board (Figure 7.13d). It keeps patients on track so that discharges happen at their correct times throughout the day.

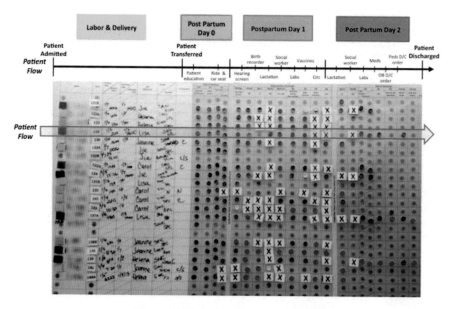

Figure 7.13d: Patient progression board

Notice that an on-time discharge starts with getting things done as early as possible in a patient's progression through the inpatient unit. In the obstetrics unit discharge board, shown in Figure 7.13d, the discharge process (planning) should start soon after admission, while the patient is on the labor and delivery service, not on the day of discharge. Although the length of stay may vary, being able to predict the day of discharge as early as possible allows us to ensure that all support services work at the expected cadence to produce an on-time and high-quality discharge, with the patient medically and socially ready.

It is important to note that the variability in the length of a stay for a given diagnosis may be minimized using clinical standardized work or a clinical pathway. This entails a timed plan of care using the best available medical evidence for the treatment of a particular condition. For the example depicted in figure 7.13, this standardized work would be post-cesarean delivery care. Clinical variability may occur, but optimally, evidence-based care will be used to decrease overall variability in the care and thus potentially in the length of the stay or the number of resources used to deliver that care.

Leveling Demand in Walk-In Clinics and Emergency Departments (EDs)

Because these areas are fed by nonscheduled patient groups, there isn't much use in trying to completely level patient flow throughout the day. Efforts have been made to smooth demand by using a sign to advertise wait times and level the discretionary input into the ED or a walk-in clinic, but this cannot address nondiscretionary patient inputs. We need to research what the demand curves look like for these operations and devise a strategy to level capacity to demand (e.g., level clinician and patient loads) by leveling demand where we can and staffing to demand where it is not level.

To get started, we need to pull historical data on when patients are coming into these services. Because demand can vary by month, season, and time of day, we suggest using anywhere from twelve to twenty-four months of data for an adequate representation.

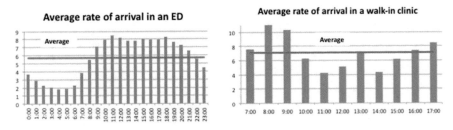

Figure 7.14: Hourly demand curves for ED and walk-in clinic

Figure 7.14 shows the futility of drawing a level loaded patient flow line (the red line) and staffing to that. Instead, we build a staffing plan that closely matches the patient demand and use a level loading box to adjust the patient flow in real time. *Heijunka* is a Japanese term for "production smoothing." The heijunka box can be a cardboard box with slots for charts or folders, or it can be computerized. Regardless of how it is set up, it is important that it can be seen by all, at a glance, so that staff and management can apportion or reprioritize the work quickly if needed.

Heijunka Box

The basic idea of a level loading box is to level areas that have large input variation so that the work can be standardized. This is done by splitting the work into short, standard time segments and loading each time slot with work that needs to be done. In the example below, thirty minutes of work equal one segment. Even though patient demand has a large variation and patients enter the system at arbitrary times, the heijunka box allows the work to be presented smoothly to the clinical staff so that high quality is maintained.

Let's say that through observation and testing we found that patient appointments in our walk-in clinic last an average of thirty minutes. As patients call for appointments, each visit is loaded as a thirty-minute work packet into a thirty-minute slot in the heijunka box, as shown in Figure 7.15 below:

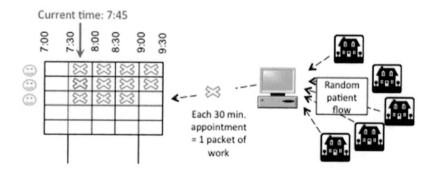

Figure 7.15: Heijunka box levels work flow

As patient demand ebbs and flows, the heijunka box visually displays the area's staffing requirements to meet the customer demand. This can be seen in the following sequences (Figure 7.16a,b).

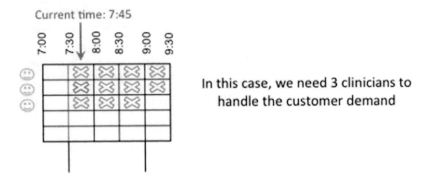

In this case, we need 3 clinicians to handle the customer demand

Figure 7.16a: Heijunka box sets necessary labor

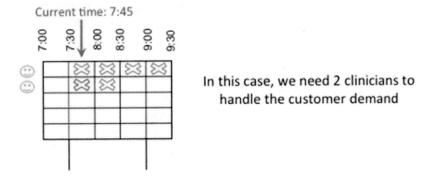

In this case, we need 2 clinicians to handle the customer demand

Figure 7.16b: Heijunka box sets necessary labor

Additionally, the maximum lead time (patient wait time) can be adjusted to meet the area's short- and long-term needs (Figure 7.16c). If staffing cannot be increased at a particular time but patient demand is increasing, the lead time can be lengthened, giving the staff consistent time to do their jobs with high quality. Conversely, if patient wait times need to decrease, adding staff will shorten the wait time while maintaining the thirty minutes needed to handle appointments with high quality (Figure 7.16d).

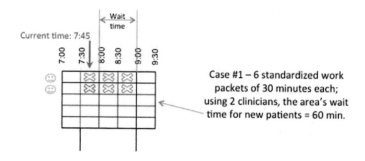

Case #1 – 6 standardized work packets of 30 minutes each; using 2 clinicians, the area's wait time for new patients = 60 min.

Figure 7.16c: Wait times can be adjusted

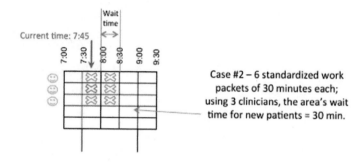

Case #2 – 6 standardized work packets of 30 minutes each; using 3 clinicians, the area's wait time for new patients = 30 min.

Figure 7.16d: Wait times can be adjusted

Another interesting aspect of the heijunka box is its ability to show the status of the area's performance in real time. If a staff member falls behind, it immediately becomes visible and stays visible until he or she is caught up (Figure 7.16e).

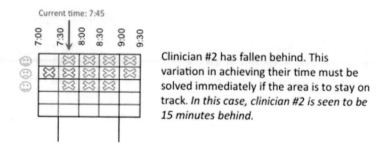

Clinician #2 has fallen behind. This variation in achieving their time must be solved immediately if the area is to stay on track. *In this case, clinician #2 is seen to be 15 minutes behind.*

Figure 7.16e: Heijunka box shows if a staff member falls behind

Because the appointments have been standardized to thirty minutes, the issues that prevent clinicians from hitting their standardized time are identified in real time. It is now management's job to help the staff by immediately eliminating issues as they appear so that the area can stay on track. This continuous improvement feature is the mechanism for better performance over time.

Using Shift Lengths as a Leveling Mechanism

When reviewing an area's demand curve, it is important to understand how shift length affects level flow. If we do nothing to change the demand, our only option is to fit capacity as closely to the demand curve as possible (Figure 7.17a).

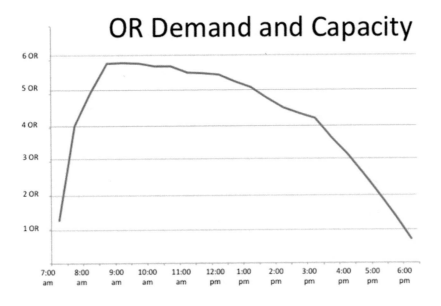

Figure 7.17a: Unleveled OR demand

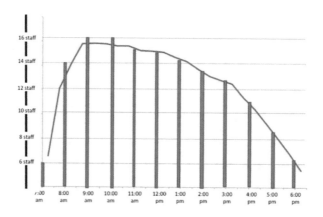

Figure 7.17b: Optimal staffing to unleveled demand

The blue bars on figure 7.17b show the optimal capacity (that is, the staffing plan) for capacity to equal demand. Unfortunately, many hospitals work twelve- or ten-hour shifts, which makes this kind of leveling impossible.

Figures 7.18a–c outline the outcome of twelve-, ten-, and eight-hour shifts. Unless the OR demand curve changes, using shift length alone to match demand and capacity creates overstaffing implications. It is clear that eight-hour shifts best minimize overstaffing.

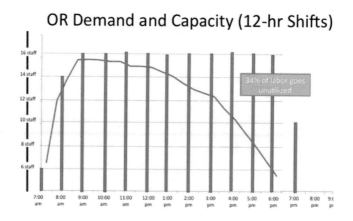

Figure 7.18a: 12 hour shift staffing to unleveled demand

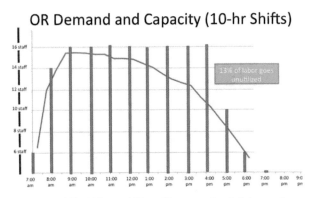

Figure 7.18b: 10 hour shift staffing to unleveled demand

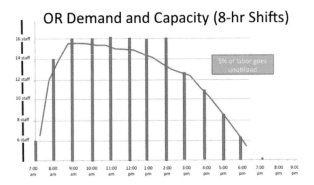

Figure 7.18c: 8 hour shift staffing to unleveled demand

Enterprise Capacity and Demand Planning

Look back at the example of how to level load an inpatient unit (Figure 7.12) and notice the strategic business decision about setting that unit's demand at twenty patients per day. That number was based on history as well as potential factors that would increase or decrease the patient census in the coming months. No one has a crystal ball, but all well run businesses need to predict future demand so that the necessary capacity is available when it is called for. To do this, top managers need to meet monthly to forecast the coming month's demand. This is called the "enterprise capacity and demand planning meeting," and it is this group's job to adjust the enterprise's cadence to what will be needed based on a forecast (Figure 7.19).

It is common to have static block schedules that set the capacity of areas like ORs. The difference with enterprise-wide capacity and demand planning is that the demand is seen as variable. Takt time is adjusted as patient demand varies from month to month so that utilization is maximized while allowing for high quality patient care and a reasonable workload for the staff.

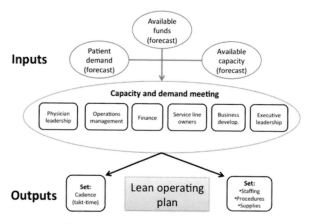

Figure 7.19: Capacity and demand planning

How to Maintain Level Flow throughout an Imperfect Day

In a real system, things are bound to get off track. Issues such as patients showing up late, supply shortages, equipment failures, and case complexity make ballet impossible unless there is a mechanism to counteract these issues as they occur. We needn't look far to find an industry that has implemented just such a mechanism: commercial aviation's air traffic control role.

Healthcare needs an air traffic or workflow control function. Critical to this function is having a patient flow lead who, like an air traffic controller, looks at patient demand and staffing capacity in real time and makes adjustments to match them. This position can be filled by a variety of people; the key to this role is the ability to see where staff members are and are not needed in real time. The workflow lead can make the most efficient use of staff and clinicians' time by moving them out of an area experiencing a lull and placing them where assistance is needed.

Implementing the Workflow Control Function

Demand and capacity leveling, or workflow control, has three requirements (Figure 7.20):

1. Enterprise capacity and demand planning, which sizes the business's capacity (and sets the takt) on a month-by-month basis

2. Level scheduling or a level discharge board, which levels the flow, hour-by-hour, on a given day

3. A workflow lead, who functions like an air traffic controller, smoothing out the inconsistencies in the day that are bound to happen; this role is supported by a workflow control manager

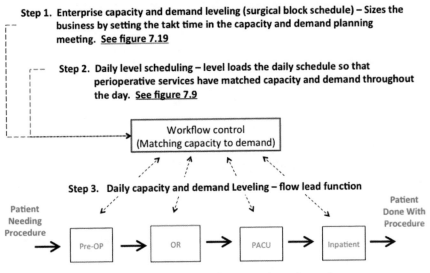

3 steps to match capacity to demand:
Perioperative services

Step 1. Enterprise capacity and demand leveling (surgical block schedule) – Sizes the business by setting the takt time in the capacity and demand planning meeting. **See figure 7.19**

Step 2. Daily level scheduling – level loads the daily schedule so that perioperative services have matched capacity and demand throughout the day. **See figure 7.9**

Workflow control
(Matching capacity to demand)

Step 3. Daily capacity and demand Leveling – flow lead function

Patient Needing Procedure

Pre-OP   OR   PACU   Inpatient

Patient Done With Procedure

Figure 7.20: Steps to matching capacity to demand

Management Requirements

Demand and capacity leveling to this degree is new in healthcare and needs a dedicated resource, which in other industries is known as "workflow control." Although there are many ways of controlling workflow in the healthcare setting, we propose that the function be made up of a workflow control manager, the scheduling team, and a workflow (or simply flow) lead.

In our hospital, the OR business manager took on the role of workflow control manager, while an experienced nurse manager took on the role of flow lead or "air traffic controller"—the only employee added to the system, because the scheduling team was already in place. These roles mitigate the "day of" variability that can occur against the leveled schedule that, in our OR example, is frozen forty-eight hours before surgery by the scheduling team. The flow lead spends 100 percent of his/her time in the work area, moving resources as needed and applying quick countermeasures to the causes of process stops in order to keep patient flow as smooth as possible. The workflow control manager supports the flow lead by spending 25 percent of his/her time in the area but has other duties such as supply chain and business analytics. This position is also instrumental in solving the root causes of the daily, recurrent issues that cause an unleveled schedule.

Executives' Role in Level Loading

No amount of improved stability can overcome an executive team that fails to incorporate monthly capacity and demand planning into its toolkit. What is the size of the business today, and what will it be tomorrow? These are not questions frontline nurses or physicians should be answering. Capacity and demand planning should not only be used to size the business today but also to understand market trends and to put resources into areas where the enterprise needs to grow.

In all lean approaches, the customer (patient) must be at the center of any business offering, so once an opportunity is uncovered in the capacity and demand meeting, it must be followed by careful study of customer requirements.

In addition to increasing understanding of the future business size and customer requirements, the capacity and demand meeting ensures that staff and clinicians will have what they need to successfully serve the future patient load.

Earlier, we examined a nurse with a fifteen-minute cycle time for patient admission who could not admit patients with high quality in less time. At the capacity and demand meeting, senior management sets the capacity so that staffing shortages are accounted for and, to the best of the business's ability, staffing is increased before shortages occur. In addition to improving patient care, this improves staff satisfaction since they are not overburdened.

CHAPTER 8

Level 4—A Takt-Driven Environment

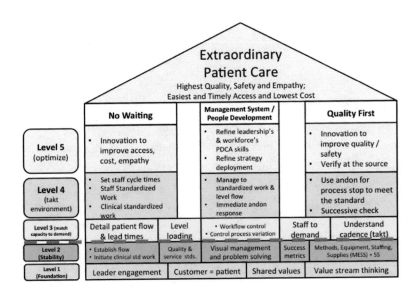

At level 1, we focused on education and alignment around the patient. At level 2, we set the stage for ballet, and at level 3, we created the cadence of the ballet (takt time). Now that we are at level 4, we can choreograph the entire cast (staff, clinicians, and managers) so that their performances lead to the same precise outcome every time. The organization's members need individual scripts that, when executed correctly, lead to *consistently* low cost and high quality outcomes. The key is consistency. High quality, low cost outcomes can occur at any level of lean, but these outputs can occur consistently only through the integration of individual scripts.

The individual scripts, which are a type of standard for how staff members do their jobs, are called standardized work. Creating standardized work is the critical first step to level 4, because it defines what processes should be followed so when there are deviations from the standard, they can be easily identified. In addition to adding standardized work, this level requires significant changes to the management structure. Clinicians and staff will not be able to follow their standards for every patient. This is why management's top priority is to keep the frontline workers on track (apply quick countermeasure problem solving) and then apply continuous improvement resources to fix the issues so that they don't stop the flow for future patients (root cause problem solving). This alignment has three requirements:

1. Manage to takt and cycle time in order to focus all support on helping the patient have the smoothest possible journey while minimizing or eliminating staff overburden.
2. Provide immediate andon response where flow stoppages exist.
3. Continuously focus on improving issues that are impeding flow via root cause problem solving.

Linking Efficiency and Quality: The Concept of Process Stop

Once a business area has been level loaded (i.e., capacity and demand are matched throughout the day), we can begin to implement no-waiting, just-in-time service (flow) with ensured quality. The link between the quality pillar and the no-waiting pillar of the lean house comes from a special feature called process stop, which must to be built into the system at this step. Process stop is analogous to line stop in manufacturing; it allows work to proceed only if the quality is correct (with a goal of perfection). If it is not, the process stops so that problems can be addressed by area management.

Taiichi Ohno famously said, "Without a standard, there can be no improvement." The idea is that once a standard exists, it is easy to see deviation from that standard. At this level of lean, when a deviation from the staff's standardized work happens, the process needs to stop and the root cause of the deviation identified so that it can be fixed and prevented.

The mechanism of process stop ensures high quality, but it seems counterintuitive that it would help with efficiency. If patient progression continually stops, fewer patients will be served, which is not the goal. To understand how process stop can benefit just-in-time service, we must remember that more than 90 percent of a typical work stream is non-value added work, much of which lies in rework, so anything that eliminates rework will greatly benefit just-in-time service for patients (Figure 8.1).

First Unit Dose for Medication on Nursing Unit

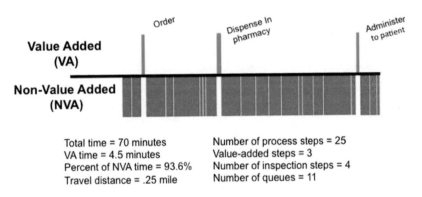

Total time = 70 minutes
VA time = 4.5 minutes
Percent of NVA time = 93.6%
Travel distance = .25 mile

Number of process steps = 25
Value-added steps = 3
Number of inspection steps = 4
Number of queues = 11

Figure 8.1: Value added / non-value added timeline

For example, when administering a medication, wasteful processes such as incorrect orders and lack of supplies on the unit require a nurse to do extra work (rework) to get to the value added job (administering the medication to the patient). With a process stop mechanism and immediate response by management to fix the issues as they occur, the patient flow is much faster than if the nurse repeatedly addresses the issues on his/her own.

As a result of rework (or work-around) cycles, systems without process stop take longer than stopping the work and fixing issues the moment they are encountered. With process stop, each patient's progression occurs with ensured quality. Over time, the processes get better, adding more value and incurring less waste due to this continuous improvement effort.

Staff and Clinician Standardized Work

Standardized work can be a confusing term, because it is often used to mean a variety of things. You may remember that in chapter 6 we showed examples of work sequences called reliable methods. "Reliable methods" and "standardized work" are often used as interchangeable terms, and until this point, that blurred definition has worked fine, though it is not entirely accurate. Now that we are building a takt-driven environment, our definition of standardized work needs to encompass four things:

1. The standardized work sequence for one frontline worker (staff or clinician)
2. The standardized supplies needed for the job outlined in that work sequence
3. Quality standards or gates that have to be met for the patient's journey to continue
4. *The standardized cycle time required to do the job outlined in the work sequence*

Note that the first three points are identical to the definition of a reliable method in chapter 6, but the fourth point, cycle time, is needed to meet the definition of standardized work. All four elements must be present. Otherwise, the work is not standardized, and level 4 work cannot be done (Figure 8.2).

There are four elements of standardized work:

1. Work Sequence – The in-order steps followed for each process
2. Standardized supplies needed for the work process
3. Quality gates that demand immediate stop and fix if quality not perfect
4. Cycle time: the time it should take to complete the work process

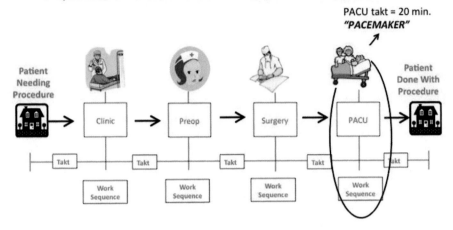

Figure 8.2: Elements of standardized work

The idea is to see where deviations from the standard occur. If we know the sequence people are supposed to follow and what supplies they will need, along with how much time the procedure should take and where or when the process should stop if quality isn't perfect, it will be easy to see where issues that block patient flow exist. The system can then be improved. The visual nature of standardized work provides management with a feedback loop when things don't go according to plan, assuming that management is readily available on the unit to receive the feedback.

Understanding Cycle Time and Patient Lead Time

Cycle time is the amount of time it takes a person or machine to do a single job. In chapter 7, we talked about a nurse whose admission process on an inpatient ward takes fifteen minutes to do properly. That fifteen-minute work cycle is called the nurse's cycle time for the admission process; it is one of the four elements of standardized work.

Cycle time must be distinguished from patient lead time, although the two are related. Patient lead time is the time the patient spends in any one area of the healthcare system (i.e., the time related to the patient care experience). As an example, patient lead time for a clinic visit could be 115 minutes, and this number would include the time it takes for a patient to park their car at the clinic, walk to the registration desk, fill out appropriate paperwork, wait prior to the examination, and receive care in the examination room. Patient lead time is related to staff cycle time in that the staff will have time-based standardized work for registering, rooming, and examining the patient. All staff cycle times, plus any waiting or transportation time, comprise the lead time that the patient experiences.

It is the function of all lean systems to decrease the non-value added time that patients experience when receiving care. As we decrease waste and support staff in meeting or improving their cycle times, patient lead times will improve. With this in mind, we will focus on understanding staff cycle time as a critical metric for a level 4 operating system. We can begin to understand the relationship between takt time, which was introduced in level 3, and cycle time, which is set and managed in level 4.

In a level 4 takt-based environment, cycle time and takt time can be used to calculate how many staff members are needed to complete work at the rate necessary to meet patient demand. For example, if it takes a nurse sixty minutes to prep a patient in the periop intake unit, we can then say that the nurse's cycle time is sixty minutes. If the takt time (patient demand rate) is twenty minutes per patient, the facility would need three nurses (60 nurse*minutes/patient ÷ 20 minutes/patient) to maintain a takt time of one patient being served every twenty minutes (Figure 8.3).

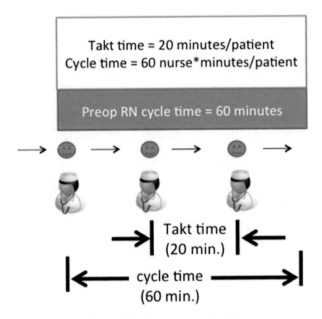

Figure 8.3: Cycle time vs. takt time

Cycle times can be used not only in one small area of a unit or service (e.g., the OR intake area) but in an entire unit or service. Figure 8.4 illustrates how to calculate staffing needs in three units of perioperative services: intake, the OR, and the PACU. The space between each patient denotes a takt time of twenty minutes per patient. As in the example above, intake needs three nurses based on the cycle and takt times. With a surgery length (cycle time) of 40 nurse*minutes/patient, two OR nurses would be needed (40 nurse*minutes/patient ÷ 20 minutes/patient). If the average stay (cycle time) in PACU is 80 nurse*minutes/patient, four PACU nurses would be needed (80 nurse*minutes/patient ÷ 20 minutes/patient).

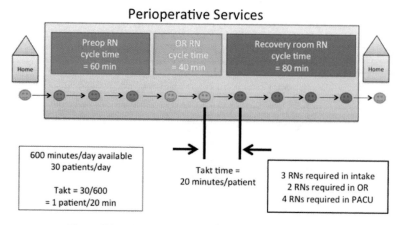

Figure 8.4: Calculating staffing using cycle and takt times

Setting Staff Cycle Times

When working with staff to set cycle times for their work, it is important for them to be comfortable with the proposed cycle times. The last thing anyone would want is for any staff member to believe the time is unattainable or feel rushed to meet it. Unfortunately, when cycle times are introduced, it is common for staff to be reticent and even angry about having time pitted against their work sequences. This is a natural reaction to a relatively new concept in healthcare, but it can be minimized.

First, it is important to explain cycle time by emphasizing that the time allotted to an individual task will be determined by the staff and clinicians themselves, not forced upon them. It has been our experience that quibbling over staff cycle times is not worth the effort as long as they are reasonable. It is far more important to set reasonable times that people believe they can meet than to have endless conversations about unfair standards. (For lean purists reading this, don't worry; as the staff become more proficient at their standardized work, cycle times will drop by virtue of the area's continuous improvement efforts. This is why we do not condone lofty cycle time targets initially.)

Second, the organization must emphasize that cycle times are never to be met at the expense of poor quality, rushing, or cutting corners. To ensure this, missed cycle times should never be addressed punitively. It is most important for management to work with staff to understand *why* the cycle time was missed, because continuous improvement will be based on the root cause(s) of the missed cycle times.

Lastly, allotting a standard cycle time to processes is a way to ensure management support. This is, at first, counterintuitive for some, but without defining a cycle time for each process, how will management know when to help? A system without time allotments risks calls for help coming too late or not at all, thus overburdening staff and leaving patients dissatisfied. The foundation of a lean system is having appropriate management leaders in the area who are ready to respond immediately to any abnormalities so that optimal patient flow can be maintained.

Choosing Easy-to-Manage Work Segments

The visual nature of standardized work allows for a feedback loop for managers, who can address issues or processes that don't go according to plan, provided that they are readily available at the unit to do so. As with all systems, the more refined the standardization, the easier it is to detect variances, so it will be important to break work sequences into small enough chunks to see issues as they occur.

Let's illustrate this concept by a hypothetical example of a process that was not broken into small enough segments. Management for an inpatient unit determined that one nurse should round on an average of three patients per hour. This statement told the nurse what the average expected rate was, but the duration of one hour and the quantity of three made it hard for anyone to see if the normal operating condition was being met while the process was underway. Additionally, because three was an average, if the nurse didn't make the expected rate, it was easy for management to assume that one patient had an unavoidable issue that made the nurse's stay run long, and thus a manager may not deem it necessary to investigate what happened. This potential lack of response to an abnormality violated the continuous improvement principle of lean.

We will need to change our approach if we want a different outcome. We need to refine the normal operating condition into short, specific quantities of time and work sequence. A level 4 management paradigm uses smaller work sequences to allow for more accurate and timely oversight and identification of abnormalities.

Breaking the work into ten- to thirty-minute segments is a good starting point (although not a hard rule). Because management expects rounding on three patients per hour, we will set the work to twenty-minute increments so that all steps of one patient's care can be completed in a cycle time of twenty minutes. Note that this new standard time *is not an average*; if the nurse gets behind during the twenty-minute cycle, immediate investigation is required.

Creating the Script: Swim Lanes

Once the staff standardized work is defined, it is important to connect the staff's standardized work to the patient's progression. (Refer to chapter 7, where patient flow was identified.)

Suppose that a patient's journey has been mapped through a perioperative services unit. The value stream in the figure 8.5 (top) demonstrates patient flow without identifying processes or patient lead times. The stream in the figure below 8.5 (bottom) demonstrates the processes that need to occur in each subunit of perioperative services.

The perioperative value stream without lead times

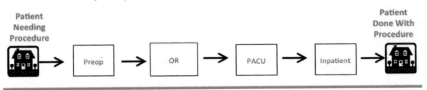

The perioperative value stream with Patient lead times

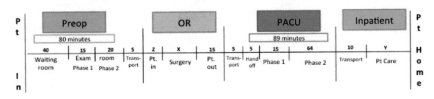

Figure 8.5: Adding lead time to the value stream map

Representing the value stream with patient lead times is an important step in choreographing the clinical staff work processes. The goal is to align the work sequences of staff and clinicians around the patient's flow. This can be done using a "swim lane" document that has patient lead times at the top (figure 8.6, narrow red oval) and individual clinical staff's cycle times added horizontally (figure 8.6, wider red oval). These map to the patient's journey through the area (in this case, perioperative services).

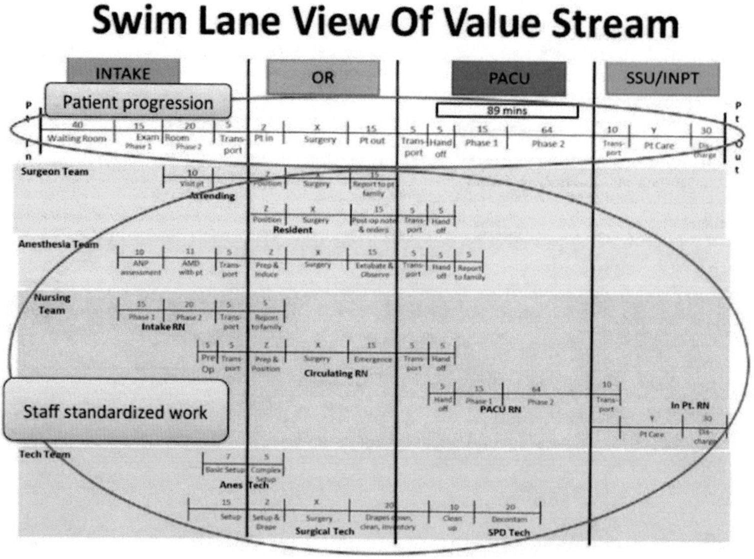

Swim Lane View Of Value Stream

Figure 8.6: Swim lane view of the value stream
(*See page 246 for expanded view of figure 8.6)

Each process has a staff member's cycle times assigned. When those times are totaled, they show the total time the patient is expected to spend in each subunit—the patient lead time. In the example above, intake lead time is eighty minutes, and PACU lead time is eighty-nine minutes. The swim lane is the script that choreographs the staff work cycles to the optimal patient flow (based on patient demand or takt). For management and staff alike, this will become the go-to document for the visual standard on patient flow as well as how to maintain the choreography that ensures smooth patient flow.

It is important to note that this is a high-level document showing cycle times for individual staff and clinician processes. It is imperative to separately document the detailed standardized work (sequence, supplies, and quality gates) that support the timed processes for each individual. In addition, a job-training matrix should document staff competency with the standardized work.

Andon: The Signal for Process Stop

In addition to refining staff and clinicians' standardized work, the organization needs to implement mechanisms to deal with imperfection. In a takt environment, imperfections show up as abnormalities from the expected operating condition. For instance, let's assume a nurse is ten minutes into a twenty-minute cycle time and has completed 25 percent of the tasks, while the standard is to complete 50 percent in ten minutes. He/she needs a way to call for help when such abnormalities occur so that he can get back on track. Andon is used for this purpose.

The term "andon" means "signal"—it is a signal to management that immediate assistance is necessary so staff and clinicians can get back to their standardized work as quickly as possible. Andons can be visual or audible—lights (Figure 8.7), bells, pages, calls, colored flags, placards on doors, or anything that area managers can readily see or hear when an issue is preventing a staff member from hitting the cycle time and thus preventing patients from continuing on their care journey.

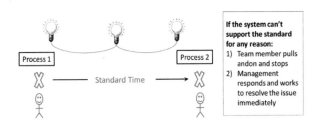

Figure 8.7: Pulling the andon

Supply shortages, absenteeism, equipment failure, and incorrect information are all examples of deviations from a standard that will need to be dealt with immediately to maintain the area's takt time. Andons should be used to call for help and get the unit back on track, in the context of quickly fixing the situation to restore patient flow (Figure 8.8). If recurring, however, the issue causing the andon should become the focus of improvement work that eliminates the root cause. This root cause problem solving can be relatively quick or can take weeks, depending on the complexity of the problem.

To maintain flow, andon and andon response must be implemented

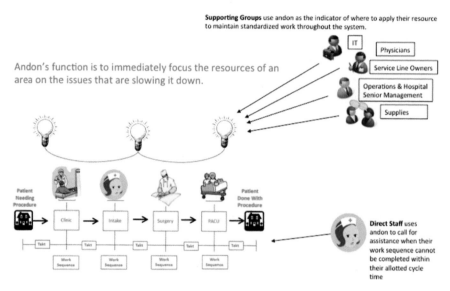

Figure 8.8: Response to andon

Team Leaders: Andon First Responders

Although many things will need to change to support a takt-driven environment, none is more important than changing management's structure and focus. The management team needs to convert from working for the levels above them to working for the levels below them. It is the leaders' primary job to enable the front line to follow their standardized work. This change cannot be overstated and will undoubtedly be the biggest stumbling block in implementing a takt-driven environment. In addition to responding immediately to andon calls by the front line, managers need to perform daily audits to ensure that standardized work is being followed and, if not, to investigate why.

In many organizations, responding to andons requires the introduction of a new leadership entity: a frontline group of process enablers commonly known as team leaders. Their work is to verify that the standardized work is being followed and the expected daily outcome is being met (Figure 8.9).

While the frontline's standardized work is kept in check by the team leaders, area management is looking at the health of the overall system. This group manages an area's overall performance to takt time by monitoring the causes of flow stoppage (andons) in each area and applying resources and help where needed. If an area shows variation, the unit management team immediately investigates and helps where needed. This is similar to a clinical arena where, for instance, a surgery cannot proceed without additional help or equipment. An immediate response enables the surgery to proceed to completion—no one would tolerate anything different. This attitude needs to extend to all processes, and the team lead role helps make that happen.

Team Leader Standardized Work

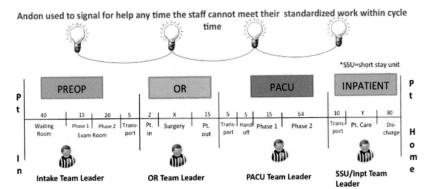

Andon used to signal for help any time the staff cannot meet their standardized work within cycle time

*SSU=short stay unit

Team Leader is responsible for the following:
1) Verify area readiness (MESS)+5S
2) Track and ensure staff are achieving their cycle time goals
3) Verify staff is following standardized work sequence correctly
4) Immediate response to andon
5) Track reasons for andon and record on the daily issues board (report these issues to management during daily gemba rounds)
6) Conduct daily improvement of the area with the staff

Figure 8.9: Team leader role

It is important to make cycle times and andons visible for all to see so that improvement efforts can be appropriately prioritized. In the cycle time and daily andon tracker tool that the team lead uses in a perioperative intake area (Figure 8.10), the cycle time standards are written at the top of the sheet. Individual nurses track their actual times, and when a cycle goes long or short, the reasons are tracked so that they can be eliminated through continuous improvement activities. Similarly, when patient flow is interrupted and an andon is used for assistance, these issues are grouped and recorded so that they can be eliminated.

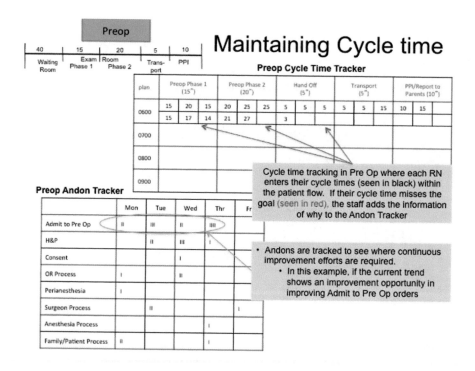

Figure 8.10: Tracking the progression of standardized work

Interplay Between the Team Lead and the Flow Lead

The flow lead (covered in chapter 7) was compared to an air traffic controller. This position's key role is to make adjustments throughout the day to make up for imperfections (variability) in capacity or demand. The flow lead maintains patient flow by moving resources to areas that need help and away from areas that don't. This person works closely with the team leader to maintain an area's on-time performance (takt time). They split the needs of a takt-driven system into two parts:

1. The team lead ensures that the area's frontline clinicians and staff can hit their cycle times.
2. The flow lead keeps a steady flow of patients coming into the area to match the area's capacity (level loading).

Because the flow lead's work is substantially predicated on the frontline staff meeting cycle times, these roles are inextricably linked (Figure 8.11).

Linkage of team leader and flow lead

Utilizing staff to maximum efficiency allows time for continuous improvement efforts in the department during working hours.

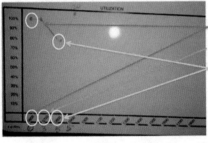

1. At 6:00 6 RNs were needed to check in first cases.
2. Once all the first cases were sent in to their procedure areas, RNs 4,5,and 6 were sent on breaks by the team lead.
3. At 8:00 the PACU needed another RN, based on the patient flow. The flow manager redeployed nurse 6 to the PACU.

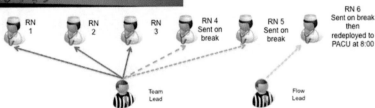

Figure 8.11: Team leader and flow lead

The "Daily" Management System in a Takt-Driven Environment

In chapter 6, we covered the fundamentals of daily management and leader standardized work. These fundamentals still apply at level 4, but in the takt-driven system, the daily feedback on problem identification is much faster. With each takt cycle comes feedback (via andon) about the issues slowing the frontline workers (and thus the patients). That means that issues affecting patient flow will potentially need to be addressed every ten to twenty minutes! This increase in problem identification needs to be met with an increase in problem resolution, which is why the management system needs to switch from *daily management* to *hour-by-hour (or minute-by-minute) management* to meet level 4 demands.

Managements' calendars at all levels need to be revised to allow for time in the gemba so that they can effectively manage the new takt-driven system. Important things to notice include the following:

1. Managers at all levels will need to reconsider their roles.
2. Each role requires more gemba time than at previous levels of lean.

Role	Time in gemba
Team lead	100 percent
Assistant nurse manager	75 percent
Manager	50 percent
Director	25 percent
CEO	10 percent

3. The requirement for andon resolution is heightened at all levels.

In practice, the daily management system is comprised of the important interactions between management and staff to monitor area cycle times and staff performance against them, as shown below (Figure 8.12).

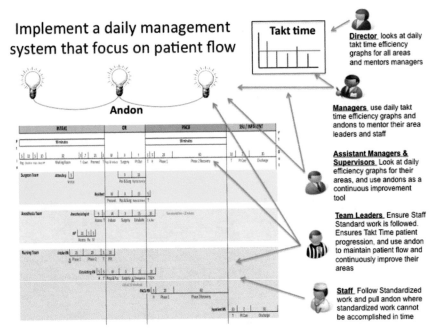

Figure 8.12: Daily management structure

Displaying Daily Efficiency

Once level 4's takt-driven environment has been implemented, real-time tracking of area efficiency can begin. Let's say that based on the swim lane diagram presented earlier (Figure 8.6), our PACU nurse's standardized work dictates that he/she should take forty-five minutes to care for one patient (fifteen minutes of phase 1 recovery, twenty minutes of phase 2 recovery, five minutes for transport, and five minutes for reporting to the patient's family).

Knowing the number of patients who should be served each hour by one nurse, the actual number of patients served, and the number of nurses available, we can calculate the area's efficiency in real time. If the intake nurse works at 100 percent efficiency, she can serve one patient every forty-five minutes (every .75 hours) or 1.33 patients per hour. Let's say that between 8:00 and 9:00 a.m., there are ten patients served and ten nurses in the area. To calculate area efficiency, we start with maximum efficiency by taking one nurse's capacity (1.33 patients per hour) and multiplying by the number of nurses: 10*1.33 = 13.3 patients to be served by all of the nurses in that one-hour period. If the actual demand is ten patients, the area's efficiency between 8:00 and 9:00 is 10 ÷ 13.3 = 0.75 = 75 percent. As the day progresses, efficiency points can be plotted each hour in real time (Figure 8.13).

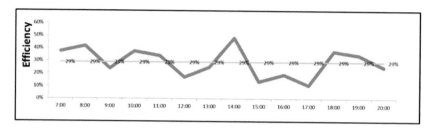

Figure 8.13: Area efficiency graph

This efficiency measure has only two elements to control: matching capacity to demand (level loading) and the staff achieving cycle times while following work sequences with perfect quality (Figure 8.14). The flow lead acts as an enabler for matching capacity to demand, and the team leader acts as an enabler for staff to meet their standardized work. Leveled demand and standardized work proficiency are thus combined to show the area's operational or takt time efficiency.

Area efficiency has two major contributing factors

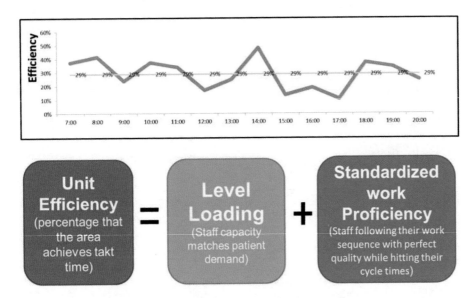

Figure 8.14: Efficiency has two components

At the outset, it is common that the work areas will be far from able to hit the takt consistently, and their efficiencies will be low. Figure 8.15 shows real data from a recovery room where a takt-driven production system was initiated. The key to improving the 29 percent efficiency rate is to understand and eliminate the issues getting in the staff's way.

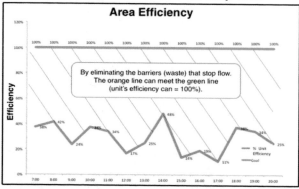

Figure 8.15: Improving efficiency

Because area efficiency is directly controlled by the staff's ability to fol-low the standardized work, every time a cycle time is not met, the reason for the stoppage is recorded, addressed, and prevented, thus increasing overall effi-ciency (Figure 8.16). This is why standardized work is such a powerful continu-ous improvement tool.

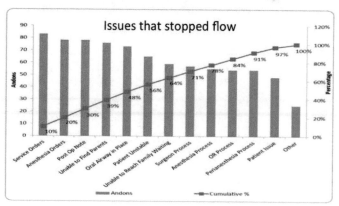

Figure 8.16: Area issues "andons"

In level 4, it is management's primary responsibility to enable frontline staff to consistently achieve their standardized work. To deal with issues in real time, a two-pronged approach is needed: 1) Team leads and the flow lead respond immediately and work on getting the flow going again (with perfect quality, as soon as possible), and 2) Management focuses continuous improvement resources on solving the issue at its root so it doesn't recur.

Becoming proficient at reliability hitting takt time will take some time; many things need to work together before it can be met reliably. In figures 8.17a–c, the area started at 29 percent efficiency (it met the takt time 29 percent of the time). As the team continuously improved level loading and cycle time performance (through waste elimination), its efficiency became 100 percent.

Performance at the beginning of level 4

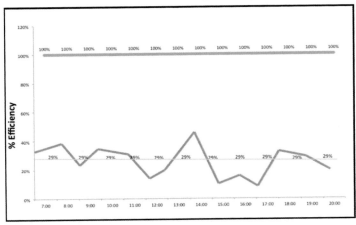

Figure 8.17a: Area before improvement

Improved matched capacity to demand and cycle time performance

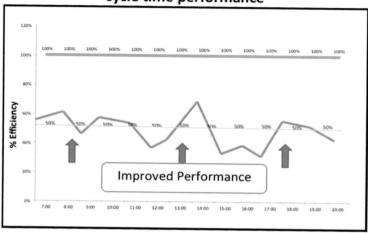

Figure 8.17b: Area with some improvement

Area Efficiency Meets Standard

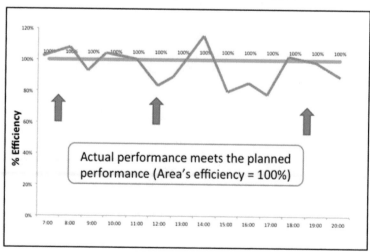

Figure 8.17c: Area that is capable of consistently achieving takt time

Measuring Performance Using the Mechanisms of an Advanced Lean System

Standardized work, andon, and daily management (managing to takt and process stop) are important advanced lean operating mechanisms that are key in moving from traditional mode (hockey) to stable processes (ballet). All three rely on each other, so they must all be present at the introduction of the takt-driven environment. In advanced lean, system stability is measured by how well team members can *consistently* achieve their cycle times. Measuring variation to planned cycle time in real time and responding to those variations allow team members to be engaged in process improvements as part of their daily work.

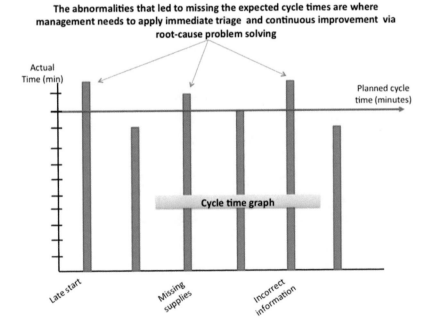

Figure 8.18: Cycle time tracking

In figure 8.18, each bar represents the actual time it took to complete the standardized task. Because the graph is produced in real time, a new bar appears as each cycle is completed. If the actual time is equal to the standard (expected time), no issue is recorded. In this case, the causes of variation (exceeding the red line "standard") are a late start, missing supplies, and incorrect information. When a variation occurs, the team lead's first order of business is to get the front line back to standard as quickly as possible so that the area can meet its overall takt time. For the late starts, the team lead might confer with the team member and ask him/her to help come up with a solution that makes it impossible to start late. In the case of missing supplies, the team lead would ask the staff member what happened and work together to prevent that issue from happening again. In the case of incorrect information, the team lead would escalate the issue to the next higher manager for help and resolve the issue so that it won't stop the area again.

Although an area may have many problems, the issues that cause measureable variation to cycle time are the most important. The goal is to solve them the same day that they occur. If left unchecked, the same issues are bound to cause measureable variations tomorrow.

The data that managers act on should be those that represent the weakest links of the daily processes so that the area becomes more capable each day. The capability of an area is the percentage of time that its actual time (the blue bars on the graph in figure 8.18) meets the expected standard time (the red line in figure 8.18) each month. Area management uses this monthly percentage, called the run ratio (Figure 8.19), to decide when the area can change the standard—this is one aspect of level 5 work (see chapter 9). The takt time performance can be tracked month over month to show how well the area is hitting its standards and ensuring smooth, high quality, timely patient flow without overburdening the staff.

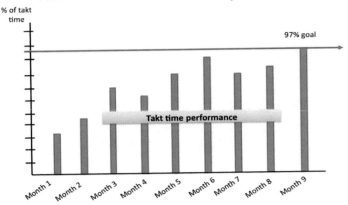

Figure 8.19: Takt time performance tracking

Typically, when an area is capable of hitting the takt time 97 percent of the time, it is time to improve the standard (more on this in chapter 9). Tracking the percentage of the time that an area meets its takt time (the run ratio) is an important measurement in a level 4 system. The graph in figure 8.20 shows a sustained run ratio of better than 97 percent for a month. This indicates that the team is ready to go on to level 5.

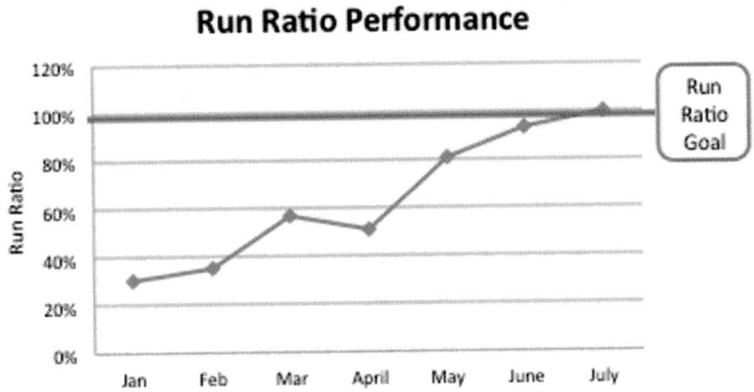

Run Ratio Performance

Figure 8.20: Run ratio performance tracking

Continuous Improvement

An understanding of level 4 work should clarify why it is critical to attain stability at level 2 before levels 3 and 4 can be properly implemented. If MESS and 5S are not consistently attained, there is no way the system can be leveled, work sequences timed, and andons managed in a timely fashion. MESS and 5S efforts are likely to reveal problems to solve. We have talked largely about the mechanisms of issue identification—how to spot problems—but not much about the mechanisms of continuous improvement that fix the problems.

The first requirement is to establish daily continuous improvement time for management, clinicians, and staff alike. We suggest one hour per day of improvement time for all team leads and managers and ten minutes per day for staff and clinicians. It is critical to have this time in place before attempting level 4 work; otherwise, the problems surfaced by the system will quickly pile up and destroy the lean effort. We also suggest forming local improvement teams that work cross-functionally to solve issues that are too large for one person to handle.

Next, align these daily improvement resources around the items that stopped flow that day. As in previous examples, most items that stop flow relate to quality, such as poor quality in the timeliness of paperwork, which will stop flow if the issues can't be resolved immediately.

It's common to implement audits to ensure high quality, yet audits have proven to be a poor mechanism to ensure quality over a long time. Audits are typically done on a small subset of processes, and the results are extrapolated to all processes. The following problems with this approach need to be fixed if we want an error-proof system:

1. Not all processes were actually audited, so even if those that *were* audited checked out okay, others might not meet the standard. Ideally, we need a system that checks *every* process, not a small subset.
2. Audits can prompt the staff to work to a higher standard while the audit is being conducted, known as "the Hawthorne Effect." We need a system that occurs naturally in the process, not as a special step.

3. Audits can evoke negative emotions in the staff. A common response is "Why are you auditing me? I know what I am doing—don't you trust me?"

A better method, which should be the focus of continuous improvement efforts in level 4, is to implement processes that eliminate the possibility of making errors in the first place.

Error-Proofing Instead of Audits

The unsatisfactory features of audits led to the invention of the successive check, a process as quick and easy to implement as it is to understand. A successive check works by engaging the next person in a process to see if the quality standards of the previous process were upheld. If not, the person doing the successive check immediately feeds the error back to the team so that it is not repeated.

An example is hand washing. Management typically audits hand-washing compliance once or twice a day. If successive checks are implemented for this process, every time caregivers meet with a patient, the first thing they verify is whether the last person who made contact with the patient washed his or her hands. If the answer is no, the abnormality is escalated to the team so that the issue does not occur again. This process could be strengthened by ensuring that staff members identify themselves by name when entering a patient's room; staff members who do not wash their hands can be identified directly and a discussion can then ensue to learn why the standard was not followed.

Successive checks are much better than periodic audits, because they check for process compliance every time the process is conducted, but the feedback is still slower than real time. In addition, many people have an adverse reaction to being checked on by others. To get around these drawbacks, the organization needs to employ the final and highest order of error-proofing: verification of quality at the source with a *poka yoke* device (poka yoke is a Japanese term that means "mistake proof"). Many devices over the years have been implemented to ensure that a quality issue cannot be passed on during the process. At this level of error-proofing, there is no need for successive checks, because the people who do the work get immediate feedback when they don't meet the quality standards.

In the hand-washing example, imagine if the door to the patient's room will not open until the incoming caregiver has washed his/her hands. This will eliminate the need for audits and successive checks.

This example suggests another characteristic of poka yoke devices: they are typically much more involved to implement. A successive check can be implemented on the same day, but a poka yoke may take days or weeks to create. The in-depth study and time required to implement source verification with poka yoke generally make this a standard approach for level 5, while quick-to-implement, successive checks are more standard for level 4.

The key phrase is "standardized approach." Although successive checks and source verification can be employed at all levels of lean, these techniques cannot be thought of as standard approaches until the unit has well-choreographed processes (level 4) or the ability to innovate (level 5). For more information on successive, source verification, and poka yoke, we refer the reader to Shigeo Shingo's book, *Zero Quality Control*.[20]

CHAPTER 9

Level 5—The Final Level
Is Not So Final

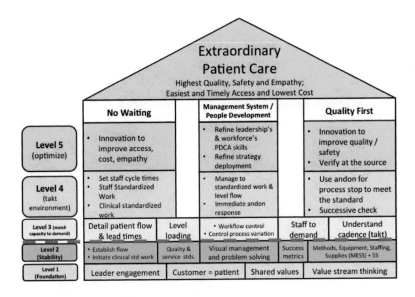

With level 4 processes in place, the lean healthcare "ballet" is choreographed and executed to a high degree by all the players. Patients flow at the expected takt time with few interruptions, quality is consistent, and access, costs, and empathy are improved. What should happen next?

In a traditional system, this would be the end of "the project." The transformation would be declared a success, and everyone would move on to other business concerns. In a lean system, this is the start. As previously stated, all operating systems are composed of at least 90 percent waste, and even the best lean transformations should expect to remove no more than 10 percent of waste as a first cut. Finding that all the efforts so far have touched "the tip of the iceberg" can be deflating. The good news is that the lean production *system,* now fully in place as a continuous improvement engine, continues to hone the organization's problem solving skills via repetitive PDCA cycles, so issues are solved at an even greater rate and level of detail than before—we are now ready to perform level 5 work. At level 5, the continuous improvement engine that was created is now used to further improve all standards, thus garnering more and more gains in quality, efficiency, and cost.

Run Ratio: A Key Continuous Improvement Mechanism

In level 4, as an area solves the quality and process issues that cause the staff and clinicians to miss their cycle times, the unit becomes more proficient at hitting its takt time until it is capable of doing so nearly 100 percent of the time. The percentage of time that an area achieves takt time is called the run ratio, which was briefly introduced in chapter 8.

> Run ratio = (the number of times an area achieves its takt time/the total number of attempts) * 100

> For example, if a unit achieves its takt time twelve times out of fifteen attempts, the run ratio = 12/15*100 = 80 percent.

Level 5 starts once an area achieves a run ratio of 97 percent or greater (Figure 9.1) for an extended period (we suggest a minimum of two weeks). At this point, many things, such as quality, staff engagement, safety, and patient lead time, can be improved, but it is important to pay special attention to quality, safety, and staff engagement as early areas of focus in level 5.

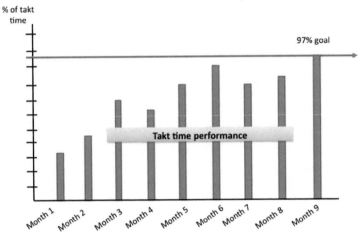

Figure 9.1: Run ratio graph

No matter what is targeted for improvement, the process follows a common PDCA cycle that continuously nets better bottom-line performance for the overall system. (To review, PDCA refers to the following: Plan = define new standardized work; Do = follow new standardized work; Check = use process stop and andon to signal management to help with the abnormalities; Adjust = implement fixes for the causes of the abnormalities that impede the new standardized work.)

Once the standardized work is updated, for example, with a new policy, it needs to be clearly communicated. Staff and clinicians should be trained on the new standard, and management should audit and support the new standard. The improvement process repeats based on how well the new standard is met.

Quality before Efficiency

As always, quality must come before efficiency. The process stop function covered in the previous chapter is the central mechanism that links process flow (time or efficiency) to process quality, so there should be a one-to-one correlation between meeting takt time and high quality. If this is not the case, the first order of business should be improving the process stop mechanism by better defining the quality standards (gates) at each step and improving management's ability to respond immediately when a process stop occurs.

Once an area's quality and flow standards are consistently met (that is, the run ratio is 97 percent or greater for an extended period), it is time to move on to improving the system beyond its initial specifications. We suggest starting level 5 improvements by improving the initial quality standards, which will affirm the key principle of quality before efficiency.

Examples of this type of improvement activity might be for a nurse on a step-down unit to round on his/her sickest patients more frequently. For instance, if the old standard was to verify a critically ill patient's condition and vital signs every twenty minutes, the new standard might be verify them every ten minutes. In this case, management and staff would change the standardized work so that the new standard could be achieved. If the new standardized work did not account for real-world issues that make the standard impossible to achieve, the increased frequency of checking vitals would give the nurse more work than he/she could handle (overburden), which would show up as a missed cycle time for the nurse. *This should not be seen as a failure*, because the system will highlight where the area is unable to meet the new standard in real time. As soon as the nurse finds that the standard cannot be met within the cycle time, he/she should invoke a process stop by pulling the andon. Management and clinicians can improve the standardized work so that it can be achieved without overburden.

Level 5 is also where verifying at the source with a poka yoke device can be used as a standard approach to ensuring quality. As noted in chapter 8, this approach stops an error from being passed to the patient by preventing the quality issue. Examples of poka yoke devices include anesthetic hoses that cannot be plugged into the wrong sockets (Figure 9.2) and doors that won't open to patient rooms until hands are properly washed.

Poka yoke
In this case gas lines in the OR cannot be connected improperly
due to each gas having a different shaped connector

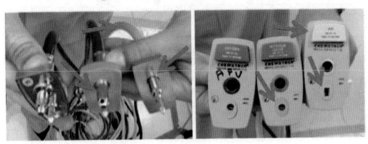

Figure 9.2: Poka yoke example

Although poka yoke devices usually take considerably more engineering than other methods of quality control, they are the highest order of ensuring perfect quality and so are well worth the effort. Although they may be employed at earlier levels, the time and lean-thinking skills needed to implement them and ensure quality throughout the system is not typically available until level 5.

Respect for Humanity

Although quality, access, cost, and service are explicitly called out as areas of improvement throughout this book, a more implicit area of improvement should not be forgotten: the area of staff engagement commonly called respect for humanity. Many things that improve flow will improve staff engagement, because making the work easier often benefits both patients and staff. Other considerations at this level have to do with staff morale more than anything else, but remember that lean systems match patient needs and staff needs to meet mutual objectives (Figure 9.3).

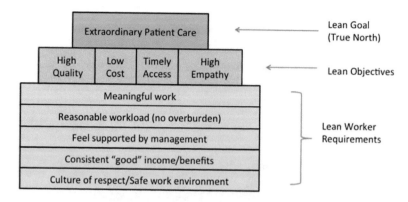

Figure 9.3: Value Proposition "mutual prosperity" between
an organization's workers and the patient

Level 5 offers the time to give extra consideration to staff and clinician engagement with improvements such as the following:

1. Improving areas where staff overburden still exists
2. Offering flexibility for people in monotonous jobs to change positions (or, better yet, eliminate the need for monotonous procedures)
3. Enhancing work area safety
4. Enhancing the culture of respect by focusing on improving working conditions

Creating an engaged team is a powerful principle of lean systems. It depends on the know-how of the entire team to solve the issues that get in the way of serving patients in the best way possible. If the team isn't highly engaged, there isn't much hope for the improvement needed to continuously improve patient care. For this reason, it's important to focus energy on team engagement.

Improvements in Cycle Time

Eventually, you will want to improve area output (efficiency) and reduce patient lead time through an area. By definition, an increase in efficiency means doing more (or the same) value added activities with fewer resources. In the takt-driven environment, efficiency gains equate to the staff doing standardized work in less time. Said another way, the cycle times in the standardized work need to be reduced. This may sound like a mechanism to ratchet up the staff's work to an even harder level, but remember that quality and staff engagement come as prerequisites to any cycle time reductions. Asking staff to work harder, stay later, and potentially cut corners is not an option.

It's important to recall the mechanisms of process stop and andon; if new cycle times cannot be met with perfect quality in a consistent and reasonable way, the process is stopped, the andon is pulled, and energy is focused on changing the process so that the staff can meet the new standard. Improving the standards (reducing cycle times or adding value added work) will uncover the next set of problems; they show up as variations to cycle time that require the team to repeat the continuous improvement process. Once these new sets of problems are abolished, the run ratio will rise above 97 percent, and the process is ready to start over again. Figure 9.4a demonstrates how, at level 4, cycle times can be consistently met so that the run ratio is attained 97 percent of the time. Figure 9.4b illustrates how changing the cycle time standard will introduce more waste or inefficiency into the system so that level 5 PDCA cycles of improvement are needed in order to reach a run ratio of 97 percent again. This cycle can be repeated in perpetuity for any number/type of work standards.

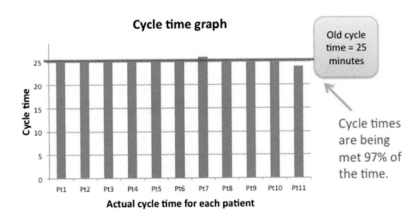

Figure 9.4a: Staff consistently hits their cycle times

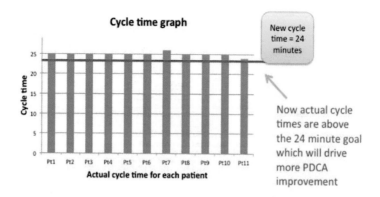

Figure 9.4b: Lower the cycle times to drive more PDCA

Using 3P as a Level 5 Improvement Methodology

Three P is a structured problem solving methodology that uses collaborative thinking to develop radical and/or innovative solutions to create the highest value care for patients. The tool helps drive revolutionary product or process design. The acronym stands for Production Preparation Process. Three P is presented in depth by Allan Coletta in his book, "The Lean 3P Advantage: A Practitioner's Guide to the Production Preparation Process", which is referenced in the bibliography.

The three P methodology represents a dramatic shift from the incremental approach of continuous improvement. To date, this book has stressed using the various principles in levels 1 through 4 to improve the existing daily work flows in healthcare. These incremental improvements to the existing work are termed kaizen improvements. Once an organization has mastered levels 1 through 4, it can now begin to innovate such that new and formerly unimagined ways of attaining work day efficiencies and quality gains that patients deserve can now be achieved. Without deeply understanding one's organizational processes (e.g. the processes optimized by level 1 through 4 work), it will be difficult for an organization to use this methodology to sustain the radically different workflow processes necessary to create the "breakthrough benefits" for patients.

Three P can be used to redesign the physical layout of the care delivery system, to create new care delivery models, or to invent new drugs or widgets for error-proofing processes. The requirements for a successful 3P approach are as follows:

1. Thorough lean understanding through levels 1 through 4
2. Thorough understanding of the process requirements based on current conditions and the desired future state.
3. Commitment to apply breakthrough thinking to problem solving by:
   a. Focusing on what must be done not what "we think" is possible
   b. Using creativity instead of capital (no extra money, no extra space, no extra people)
   c. Going to alternate sources such as nature to find inspiration for improved solutions
4. Use try storming over brain storming:
   a. Each member of the 3P team needs to come up with 7 different new process designs
   b. Each design is thoroughly reviewed and tested as a prototype in actual operations. Thus, rapid testing of the ideas in an actual production area (try storming) is used rather than discussing in a meeting room (brain storming)
   c. Combine all successful ideas into one new process and rapidly implement into production
5. Repeat the process anytime major gains need to be made

Thinking and Acting Differently in Level 5

Albert Einstein famously said, "We cannot solve our problems with the same level of thinking that created them." Under this logic, the level 5 organization will need to significantly improve its ability to innovate in order to eliminate process waste that it has not been able to remove. This shift will require management, clinicians, and staff at all levels to reorganize how they engage in improving the gemba—which, when viewed through a traditional lens, may seem peculiar. For example, at level 5, the following issues may need to be addressed:

1. Executives recognize that they need to be much closer to what is going on, so they move their desks out of their offices and into the gemba.

2. Managers are rewarded for eliminating unnecessary meetings and email so they can speed improvements by spending nearly all day on process improvement activities in their areas.

3. Physicians, nurses, staff, and management all have the same alignment and incentives (without exception), that focus on continuously improving the patient care experience.

4. Every staff member makes a process improvement every day, which requires each staff member and clinician to spend a portion of every day in structured, continuous improvement. If there are one hundred people in an area, the expectation becomes one hundred improvements per day.

5. The staff members push for operational efficiency gains, because they understand that the efficiency of the overall system benefits them personally through a heightened sense of mission, no overburden, a culture of respect, a safe work environment, job security, and good pay.

6. The total patient lead time is reduced by more than 50 percent through continuous reduction in staff cycle times and patient wait times.

7. Total quality issues are reduced by more than 50 percent through continuous improvement of quality standards and implementing of source verification.

8. Executives become emboldened by "seeing with their own eyes" the effects of an advanced lean system, and make the spread of advanced lean a core goal for the organization.

These examples are the tip of the iceberg once level 5 takes hold in an organization. Einstein also said, "We must act differently to produce different results."

CHAPTER 10

Putting It All Together

We hope that this book helps healthcare leaders move a step closer to transforming their organizations into an advanced lean system. The key is to start the transformation as soon as possible and to be willing to make corrections as you go rather than waiting for the perfect plan. There is no such thing as a perfect lean implementation plan, so putting off the start date until one exists will only delay your organization's progress. The lean mindset dictates that learning by trying is more important than analyzing and waiting for the "right" moment.

As your lean effort builds momentum, you will learn more about lean by *doing* than any book can teach. As your learning continues, the levels of an advanced lean implementation will become clearer, so don't spend too much time trying to understand the nuances of the advanced levels if you are just beginning.

Here is a review of a few key points for each level of a lean transformation.

Level One: The Foundation

Outline your organization's true north alignment. It should center on the needs of the patient, the company, and its people, and this alignment will be used to measure "Are we doing the right things?" from this point forward. Also, this true north message needs to be communicated to the entire organization so that the goals—what a successful lean transformation will look like—are known by all.

Start implementation by aligning the senior leaders (administrative as well as clinical) around any one of a number of patient flows, and then create a shared vision of what your future state lean organization could look like. It is critical to align and engage senior leaders at this phase; until that is complete, it will be impossible to align and engage other levels of the organization.

Construct a lean resource team that will help your organization work through the details. These resources should include a process improvement team as well as external senseis for deep lean knowledge. Partner these resources with your human resources and/or organizational development teams to help with change management. This partnership reduces the risk that the lean work will be seen as a project, separate from how you run your organization day-to-day.

Once this initial alignment is attained, identify a "burning platform" driver and build an A3 diagram outlining the current state and proposed improvements, addressing questions like "Why we are doing this?" As a team, create a vision of perfect quality with the ideal customer and staff experience and which uses the fewest resources possible. Pick a place to start that moves your organization one step closer to your vision. Ideally, your initial project should highlight the importance of looking at flow in the context of a value stream. For example, you could start by creating a value stream map of the cardiac program, from the referral process to outpatient visits to inpatient admissions that encounter perioperative services, and then to the intensive care unit, the acute care ward, the rehabilitation facility, and home follow-up.

Level Two: Stability

This level is all about creating operational stability. Experience shows that in a typical healthcare organization, this stage may take several years. Stability can be accomplished by running multiple improvement events focused on stabilizing methods, equipment, staffing, and supplies (MESS) as well as implementing the daily management and problem solving skills that will be needed to sustain the improvements.

This is the stage where most of the frontline staff gets involved in the lean improvement effort. Activities such as 5S events, kanban implementation, visual management systems, and preventive equipment maintenance improvement events all work to improve the ability of staff members in the area to do their work, albeit with largely unchanged overall workflows. A common approach is to aggressively pursue stability in a model or learning line. Consider devoting significant process improvement and sensei resources to working with this line. This is not a proof of concept, since the concept has been proven in many other places. Rather, it demonstrates how to make lean work in your culture and provides lessons for the rest of the organization to learn from, as each department or group will go only as fast as its local conditions allow.

Level Three: Match Capacity to Demand (Transition to Ballet)

Level three is where an advanced lean transformation begins. Moving to this stage is a big leap for any healthcare organization. At this stage, the tempo of the work area is smoothed by continuously matching capacity to demand. This is done by implementing new scheduling methodologies and a new management entity—workflow or production control. Level three's goal is to level the patient flow where possible and move staff flexibly where variable demand exists in order to allow staff to work at a consistent pace. It is at this level that the staff begins to experience less chaotic workloads and the patients begin to spend less time waiting for care.

Level Four: Takt Environment

Once stability is reached (Level 2) and capacity is matched to demand (Level 3), the staff and their managers will be capable of implementing a takt environment in an area. This is accomplished by introducing staff standardized work—with process stop—as well as another new management entity, the team lead. The team lead's standardized work is principally to immediately respond to andons that are stopping key processes and to perform daily improvements. The requirement to fix all issues that stop patient, material, staff, information, or equipment flow will dramatically increase the need for daily, even immediate, problem solving by management and staff. In turn, these mechanisms will make it possible to maintain patient flow to a takt time, with perfect quality.

Level Five: Optimize

Finally, as the area becomes proficient at meeting its patient flow target to a takt time with perfect quality, area staff will need to continuously improve their work by optimizing quality or patient flow standards. This never-ending process continues in perpetuity.

Johnny's Story Reimagined in an Advanced Lean System

To broaden our view of what might be possible in healthcare, let's revisit the story of Johnny that was presented in chapter 1.

This time, we imagine that Johnny's care is delivered in the setting of an advanced lean healthcare system. The system is adept at performance improvement, and many of the principles and practices outlined in this book are in place. Healthcare provision is not perfect, but the differences in Johnny's experience of care are apparent.

It's a Sunday morning in August, and while most children are enjoying the final weeks of their summer break, an eight-year-old boy named Johnny is waking up in a hospital bed. He has been battling cancer for many months, and his disease has progressed; there is no hope for a cure.

Over the last two months, his outpatient care team of physicians, nurses, and care navigators has had several gut-wrenching discussions with his family, and his care goals were transitioned to palliative care several weeks ago. (Per the hospital's standard, these difficult discussions are now facilitated by the outpatient team to help families make informed decisions.)

Johnny is nearing the end of a week-long hospital admission that began with uncertainty over whether he would survive. As fortune would have it, Johnny's condition has stabilized over the past week, and he is much more comfortable.

During family-centered rounds this morning, the discussion has turned to preparing for Johnny's discharge. (The standardized lead time for complex discharge preparation is forty-eight hours). Using an on-site Spanish interpreter, the inpatient team is running through the progress on Johnny's medical problem list and the discharge preparation checklist with his mother, his case manager, and his nurse. A multidisciplinary team performs this clinical standardized work and successive quality checks.

Johnny's mother has appreciated participating in rounds each morning, and she has her list of questions ready. Anticipating this discussion and the need to use a Spanish interpreter, Johnny's inpatient care team level loaded their work by scheduling an appointment with Johnny and his mother that is twenty minutes longer than usual for this morning's rounds. The plan is to transfer Johnny to an inpatient facility specializing in pediatric hospice care. The team predicts that Johnny will be ready for transfer on Tuesday, and it wanted to update his family and confirm that they prefer inpatient hospice care.

As per the standard, the team communicates to Johnny and his mother that while it can't be certain he will be ready on Tuesday, the discharge date prediction accuracy at forty-eight hours is about 80 percent. Everyone agrees to plan for a Tuesday discharge, and an 11:00 a.m. discharge time is targeted and posted for visual management.

Johnny's mother has two concerns she wants addressed. First, at the time of his admission, the care providers noted that Johnny's G-tube was leaking. Dealing with this issue was deferred because of more pressing concerns, but yesterday, because Johnny continued to recover, the team resurfaced the issue. His mother wants the leak to be addressed, because it bothers him occasionally. Generally, this issue is handled by placing a tube of a slightly larger diameter, which takes only a few minutes.

The second issue is that Johnny's home-feeding formula was changed to an inpatient formula during his stay, and at the time of discharge, his mother wants him to switch back to his regular formula, which she notes that he tolerates better.

To address the G-tube leak, those on the medical team need to consult with their gastroenterology colleagues. The team knows that a nonurgent G-tube change won't happen until the next day, but it notifies the gastroenterology service of the nonurgent consultation need anyway, because this is the new process it is using.

Over the past few months, many andons have been triggered by the consultation process. Several iterations of the PDCA cycle have been made to the standardized work processes for placing nonurgent consultation requests across the hospital, including whether to place nonurgent consultation requests in the late afternoon and on weekends. The new process is to place the consultation request in the computer when the decision is made, and the consulting service is automatically and immediately notified. It took a dedicated work group four weeks to design a reasonable automated notification process, but now that the new standard has been created, the notifications are going through to the consulting service's encrypted smartphone. During the day, the team can expect the consultant fellow to call back within thirty minutes. When a request is placed overnight, it is handled the next morning unless it is labeled urgent (per the new standard).

After a brief discussion, the gastroenterology consultant examines his workload, determines that his team will be by at 9:00 a.m. the next morning, and books the consultation into the patient's calendar. It has been an unusually busy week for the gastroenterology service, so all three of their Monday morning consult slots, which were created to level their workload, are taken—this happens only about once every ten days. The fellow who followed the established overbooking method (for matching staffing to demand) can see that several gastroenterology clinic appointments are open in the outpatient clinic across the street. She blocks off a clinic appointment so that the clinic fellow, who is cross-trained, can accommodate Johnny's inpatient consult. G-tube changes of this sort generally take less than thirty minutes, so there are no anticipated issues with getting things set for Johnny prior to his discharge on Tuesday.

By the end of the day on Sunday, the care team has completed its discharge preparation checklist. Tasks are clearly delineated between the physicians, case managers, and nurses. Despite the complexity of the discharge, the patient care team feels confident that everything will proceed smoothly.

At 9:00 a.m. on Monday, the gastroenterology fellow evaluates Johnny and notes an issue when preparing the G-tube change: the hospital doesn't stock the particular G-tube in the size that Johnny needs. The fellow initiates an andon, calls the materials management supervisor, and explains the problem. The need for a nonstocked G-tube happens rarely (about once every few months, which is why one is not available in the standard kanban supply system), but the team lead immediately responds to the andon. Within minutes, the team lead contacts the *hospital supply supervisor. This escalates to an outside vendor associated with the hospital that has a larger selection of tubes; it is contacted to courier the tube over within two hours.*

The lack of the needed supply is logged, as always, for ongoing analysis regarding which supplies are appropriate to stock to ensure stable supplies for patients. Moreover, the materials supervisor notifies his manager (using an andon), because the central supply department is supposed to be notified twenty-four hours ahead of the need for a nonstocked item. As the first step in solving the problem, the manager talks to the gastroenterology team later in the day to uncover why there wasn't advanced warning.

Meanwhile, the fellow has to book a time to come back and replace the G-tube later in the day. She notifies her medical director about the issue (using an andon), because several schedules are affected. Later in the day, it is discovered that a step in the process was skipped when the G-tube change was booked, which kept materials management out of the loop. The medical director and materials manager plan to sit down the next day to figure out how to solve the root cause and error-proof the process.

When the care team rounds with Johnny and his mother at 10:00 a.m. on Monday, they confirm that he is progressing as expected medically and that his discharge plan remains appropriate (representing a successive quality check). In addition to the G-tube change, the team discusses Johnny's discharge medications and feeding formula. Because perfect communication and information flow are not supported by siloed care management, the case manager and bedside nurse are part of the conversation, and preparations are made for transportation at the time of discharge and communication with the inpatient hospice facility.

On Monday afternoon, using the electronic health record (EHR) system, it takes forty-five minutes to reconcile Johnny's thirteen medications, and the physician sends the prescriptions electronically to the outpatient pharmacy. The physician calls the pharmacy to let it know that the prescriptions are all Johnny's medication for his discharge at 11:00 a.m. on Tuesday (per the standardized method). Having to make the call is frustrating, but multiple experiments and process failures have demonstrated that a call dramatically improves the pharmacy's ability to prepare medications in a timely fashion. Ideally, this phone communication could be done electronically when entering the prescriptions, but the technology isn't presently versatile enough.

The hospital's chief medical officer, who is helping to solve this big problem, has contacted the EHR company twice in the last month to provide feedback on the difficulties encountered with entering prescriptions and communicating anticipated discharge times. Because prescription entry is often the cause of patient delays, plans are underway to implement an intermediate countermeasure: employing pharmacy technicians to help electronically enter discharge prescriptions to offload the physician overburden. The hospital IT department has a standing task force (a local improvement team) that is looking for a better long-term solution.

As the pharmacy staff try to fill the prescriptions, they note that a particular medication is not available. While the other medications are being prepared, the pharmacy is easily able to identify the attending physician from the medical record and pages her while she is in the clinic. Because she is on service, her clinic day has several built-in ten-minute breaks that allow her to answer pages expeditiously. An alternate medication is chosen.

In preparing for Johnny's transfer, the case manager prepares his discharge transportation and transfer communications according to the standardized workflow process. After running through her checklist, she is reminded that Johnny will need a "Do Not Resuscitate" order signed for his transportation. This physician order, which is appropriate for Johnny's care, instructs the paramedics not to attempt resuscitation if Johnny's breathing or heart stops during transport. The case manager prepares the order and has it ready for the physician to sign. The case manager arranges for a phone call between the primary care team member and the accepting hospice physician so that an appropriate hand-off can occur.

In the meantime, the primary care team member is finishing the summary note about the patient's stay. Much of the note has already been prepared, because keeping it updated is part of the standardized work for each patient's care. Usually, this note only needs to be completed within twenty-four hours of discharge, but because Johnny is transferring facilities, it must be completed prior to his discharge. Because the case manager was present on rounds, and she follows a standard discharge check sheet for all patients, she is easily able to remind the team of the requirement.

By the end of the day on Monday, Johnny's discharge plan is set, and if he continues to be medically stable, he will be ready for transfer in the morning.

On Tuesday at 10:00 a.m., the care team is finished rounding, and Johnny is ready for discharge. Because his situation is complex, a full hour has been scheduled for the bedside nurse and case manager to review his discharge quality gates. From 10:00 to 11:00 a.m., his medications, care instructions, and medical records are reviewed. All of his mother's questions are answered without rushing. Verification of hand-off to the accepting facility occurs, and at 11:00 a.m., Johnny leaves the hospital to take what is likely his last car ride.

In this version of the story, there is much better planning and much less frustration. The care delivered from this system looks less like a hockey game and more like ballet. In the lean system careful attention has been given to designing and choreographing care processes and even greater attention is paid to times when a process fails. Frontline providers to quickly identify and fix issues while continuing to provide care for other patients with much less overburden or chaos. Managers and supervisors are aware of issues and help to solve the problems at their root cause. The system is far from perfect, but there is great internal capability for improvement.

This is what a high quality, safe, affordable, continuously improving, proactive healthcare organization might look like. It is a system worthy of the staff members who have dedicated their lives to serving patients and worthy of the patients who place in the system their sacred trust.

Notes

Chapter 1

1. Rother M. Toyota Kata: Managing People for Improvement, Adaptiveness, and Superior Results. New York, NY: McGraw Hill, 2009.

Chapter 2

2. Kohn LT, Corrigan J, and Donaldson MS. To Err Is Human: Building a Safer Health System. Washington, D.C.: National Academy Press, 2000.

3. Landrigan CP, Parry GJ, Bones CB, Hackbarth AD, Goldmann DA, Sharek PJ. Temporal trends in rates of patient harm resulting from medical care. New England Journal of Medicine. 2010; 363(22): 2124–2134.

4. Classen DC, Resar R, Griffin F, et al. "Global trigger tool" shows that adverse events in hospitals may be ten times greater than previously measured. Health Affairs. 2011; 30(4): 581–589.

5. Berwick DM, Hackbarth AD. Eliminating Waste in US Health Care. Journal of the American Medical Association. 2012; 307(14):1513-1516.

6. Womack JP, Jones DJ, and Roos D. The Machine That Changed the World. New York, NY: Harper Perennial, 1991.

7. Institute of Medicine (U.S.). Crossing the Quality Chasm: A New Health System for the 21st Century. Washington, D.C.: National Academy Press, 2001.

8. Facts about the National Patient Safety Goals. The Joint Commission WebSite.http://www.jointcommission.org/facts_about_the_national_ patient_safety_goals/ Updated July 15, 2014. Accessed July 22, 2014.

9. McCannon CJ, Hackbarth AD, Griffin FA. Miles to Go: An Introduction to the 5 Million Lives Campaign. Joint Commission Journal on Quality and Patient Safety. 2007; 33(8): 477–484.

10. Riess H, Kelley JM, Bailey RW, Dunn EJ, Philips M. Empathy Training for Resident Physicians: A Randomized Controlled Trial of a

Neuroscience-Informed Curriculum. Journal of General Internal Medicine. 2012; 26: 1280–1286.

Chapter 4

11. Sirolli E. "Want to Help Someone? Shut Up and Listen: Learning from the Hippos." TED talk. http://www.ted.com/talks/ernesto_sirolli_want_to_help_someone_shut_up_and_listen Published September 2012. Accessed April 2014.

Chapter 5

12. Reason J. Human error: models and management. British Medical Journal. 2000; 320: 768–70.

13. Hallet M. "Opening the Door of Lean to Physicians." Webinar. http://members.healthcaevalueleaders.org/page/webinars-1. Published June 26, 2013.

14. Billi J. "Engaging Physicians to Solve Real Problems in Healthcare." The Lean Post. http://www.lean.org/leanpost. Published June 24, 2013. Accessed April 16, 2014.

15. Shook J. Managing to Learn: Using the A3 Management Process. Cambridge, MA: Lean Enterprise Institute; 2008.

16. Marksberry P, Bustle J, Clevinger J. Problem solving for managers: a mathematical investigation of Toyota's 8-step process. J Manuf Technol Manag. 2011; 22(7): 837–52.

17. Nelson EC, Batalden PB, Huber TP, et al. Microsystems in health care: Part 1. Learning from high-performing front-line clinical units. Joint Commission Journal on Quality Improvement 2002; 28(9): 472–493.

Chapter 6

18. WHO Surgical Safety Checklist. http://www.who.int/patientsafety/safesurgery/ss_checklist/en/index.html. Published May, 2008. Accessed March 3, 2014.

19. Wakamatsu Y. The Toyota Mindset: The Ten Commandments of Taiichi Ohno. Bellingham, WA: Enna Inc; 2009.

Chapter 8

20. Shingo S. Zero Quality Control: Source Inspection and the Poka-Yoke System. New York, NY: Productivity Press; 1986.

Bibliography

Baker M, et al. Making Hospitals Work: How to Improve Patient Care while Saving Everyone's Time and Hospital's Resources. Cambridge, MA: Lean Enterprise Academy; 2009.

Bicheno J, and Holweg M. The Lean Toolbox: The Essential Guide to Lean Transformation, 4th ed.

Rosebank, Johannesburg: Production and Inventory Control, Systems and Industrial Engineering Books; 2009.

Coletta A. The Lean 3P Advantage: A Practitioner's Guide to the Production Preparation Process. New York, NY: Productivity Press, 2012.

Graban M. Lean Hospitals: Improving Quality, Patient Safety, and Employee Engagement, 2d2nd ed. New York, NY: Productivity Press, 2011.

Hirano H. 5S for Operators: 5 Pillars of the Visual Workplace. Productivity Press Development Team, 1996.

Jones D, and Womack J. Seeing the Whole Value Stream, 2nd ed. Cambridge, MA: Lean Enterprise Institute; 2011.

Kenney D. Transforming Health Care: Virginia Mason Medical Center's Pursuit of the Perfect Patient Experience. New York, NY: Productivity Press; 2012.

Liker JK, and Meier D. The Toyota Way Fieldbook. New York, NY: McGraw-Hill; 2005.

Liker JK and Convis GL. Toyota Way to Lean Leadership: Achieving and Sustaining Excellence through Leadership Development. New York, NY: McGraw-Hill; 2011.

Mann D. Creating a Lean Culture: Tools to Sustain Lean Conversions, 2nd ed. New York, NY: Productivity Press; 2010.

Protzman C, et al. Leveraging Lean in Healthcare. New York, NY: CRC Press; 2011.

Rother M, et al. Learning to see: Value Stream Mapping to Add Value and Eliminate MUDA. Cambridge, MA: Lean Enterprise Institute; 1999.

Shook J. Managing to Learn: Using the A3 Management Process. Cambridge, MA: Lean Enterprise Institute; 2008.

Smalley A. Creating Level Pull. Cambridge, MA: Lean Enterprise Institute; 2009.

Toussaint J, and Gerard R. On the Mend: Revolutionizing Healthcare to Save Lives and Transform the Industry. Cambridge, MA: Lean Enterprise Institute; 2010.

Wellman J, et al. Leading the Lean Healthcare Journey: Driving Culture Change to Increase Value. New York, NY: Productivity Press; 2011.

Womack JP and Jones DT. Lean Thinking: Banish Waste and Create Wealth in Your Corporation, 2nd ed. New York, NY: Productivity Press; 2003.

Womack J. Gemba Walks, 2nd ed. Cambridge, MA: Lean Enterprise Institute; 2011.

Toussaint, J. and R. Gerard. *On the Mend: Revolutionizing Healthcare to Save Lives and Transform the Industry.* Cambridge, MA: Lean Enterprise Institute, 2010.

Womack, J. P. and D. T. Jones. *Lean Thinking: Banish Waste and Create Wealth in Your Corporation,* 2d ed. New York: Productivity Press, 2003.

Womack, J. *Gemba Walks,* 2d ed. Cambridge, MA: Lean Enterprise Institute, 2011.

	Leadership Triangle	Executive Objectives	Senior Manager Objectives	Area Manager Objectives	Staff & Clinician Objectives
Level 5		• Mature demand and capacity planning • Coach in gemba enterprise-wide	• Continuous improvement via cycle time reduction • Daily continuous improvement • Implement error proofing	• Manage cycle time reduction • Daily improvement with staff against issues that impede flow • Implement error proofing	• Adhere to standardized work • Andon when standardized work cannot be met • Root-cause solve issues that impede flow
Level 4		• Enterprise-wide goal, deployment mature • Continue gemba rounds (coach in VS and help staff fix problems)	Implement: • Immediate andon response • Standardized work • Efficiency graphs assessment	• Implement team lead • Immediate andon response • Verify standardized work adherence • Efficiency graphs to manage pt. flow	• Adhere to standardized work • Andon when standardized work cannot be met • Root-cause solve issues that impede flow

Level 3		• Implement VS demand and capacity planning
		• Understand VS, takt
		• Continue gemba rounds
			• Calculate takt
			• Implement production control
			  • Capacity & demand planning
			  • Level scheduling
			  • Air traffic control
				• Staff to leveled schedule (day before)
				• Adjust staffing to actual demand (day of)
					• Staff begins to feel more consistent workload

Level 2		• Begin managing by VS • Help solve issues in the gemba	• Patient flow owned by one entity (senior mgr.) • Senior mgr.'s primary responsibility is to fix all issues that impede patient flow • Coach in the gemba	• Coach in the gemba • Maintain MESS • Shift from managing people to managing processes • Respond to staff issues	• Staff feels mgmt.'s presence • Support through MESS improvements • Begin to surface issues with daily work
Level 1		• Study trips & lean education • Go see issues • Customer (value stream) alignment	• No value stream (patient flow) alignment • Groups managed in silos by lines of authority	• Daily work largely driven by MBO requirements • Respond to area emergencies (triage)	• Staff feels minimal support from mgmt. • Limited ability to improve area

240

Consistent Patient Experience	Easiest Access	Highest Quality	Lowest Cost	Highest Empathy
Level 5	• Shortest wait times and fastest service through continuous lead time improvement	• Highest quality stemming from increasing amount of error proofing (i.e., source inspection)	• Lowest overall system cost through continuous cycle time improvement (~30%) • Significant opportunity to pass savings onto customer	• Highest level of compassion through continuous improvement of standard (courtesy, respect, listening, responsiveness, special touches)
Level 4	• Additional decrease in wait times due to following standardized work and meeting takt	• Significant increase in quality from building quality into staff standardized work: • Consistent processes • Line stop • Self-inspection	• Continue to significantly reduce overall system cost (~30%) • Growing opportunity to pass savings to customer	• Build empathy into staff standard work resulting in higher levels of : • Courtesy • Respect • Listening • Responsiveness
Level 3	• Significant decrease in wait times due to: • Capacity and demand planning • Level scheduling • Air traffic control	• Increased quality via: • Consistent cadence, allowing time for staff to focus on patient	• Begin to significantly reduce overall system cost (~10%) • Opportunity to pass savings to customer	• Increased opportunity for empathy and special touches via a consistent cadence, allowing time for staff to focus on patient
Level 2	• Slightly decreased wait times due to improved: • Staffing • Scheduling • Fewer barriers via VS alignment • Language • Transportation	• Quality slightly increased via: • Quality gates • Audits • Work standards	• Reduce overall system cost slightly (~5%)	• Slightly increased opportunity for compassion and special touches via: • DMS • Problem solving • Visual management
Level 1	• System inconsistency results in long wait times • Scheduled appts. • Waiting room • Transportation difficulties • Language barriers	• System inconsistency results in high occurrence of : • HAI's • Medical errors • Incorrect information • Poor handoffs • Many work-arounds	• System inconsistency results in high cost • Service is too expensive	• System inconsistency results in lack of: • Courtesy, respect, listening, responsiveness • No time for special touches

	Quality / Safety	Stabilize MESS	Matching Capacity to Demand	Standard Work & Andon Response	Optimize the Standard
Level 5	Mistake proof (Process Stop)				• Mistake proofing or poka yoke can be implemented as a standard practice through process redesign
Level 4	Self-inspect (Process Stop)			• Quality steps are built into standardized work • Process stop is in place • Management enables staff by responding and helping with issues	• No change to system
Level 3	Unit inspects	• Process stabilization and visual management	• Staffing matched to demand allows the area to consistently inspect due to proper staffing levels	• No change to system	• No change to system
Level 2	Inspect @ discharge	• No change to system	• No change to system	• No change to system	• No change to system
Level 1	Patient inspects	• No change to system	• No change to system	• No change to system	• No change to system

	Cost Reduction	Stabilize MESS	Matching Capacity to Demand	Standard Work & Andon Response	Optimize the Standard
Level 5	45%	(arrow)	(arrow)	(arrow)	• Area standards are redesigned to operate much more efficiently
Level 4	30%			• Staff works to a timed standard • Management enables staff to meet their standard every patient	• No change to system
Level 3	10%		• Staffing matched to demand (no extra staffing)	• No change to system	• No change to system
Level 2	5%	• No searching or waiting for supplies, equipment	• No change to system	• No change to system	• No change to system
Level 1	0%	• No change to system			

Lean Levels	Leadership / Staff	Cost Reduction	Quality / Safety	Consistent Patient Experience
Level 5		45%	Mistake proof — Process Stop	
Level 4		30%	Self-inspect — Process Stop	
Level 3		10%	Unit inspects	
Level 2		5%	Inspect at discharge	
Level 1		0%	Patient inspects	

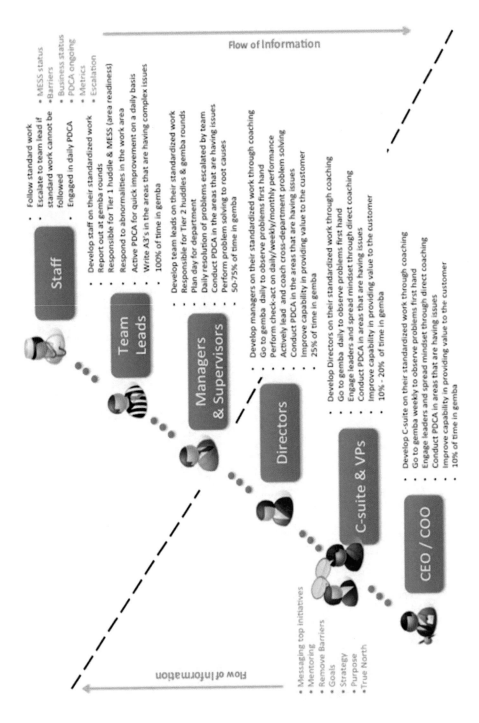

Swim Lane View Of Value Stream

INTAKE	OR	PACU	SSU/INPT

Patient progression

89 mins

Waiting Room — 40 | Exam Room Phase 1 — 15 | Phase 2 — 20 | Trans-port — 5 | Pt In — 2 | Surgery — X | Pt out — 15 | Trans-port — 5 | Hand off — 5 | Phase 1 — 15 | Phase 2 — 64 | Trans-port — 10 | Pt Care — Y | Dis-charge — 30

Surgeon Team

Visit pt — 10 | **Attending** | Position — 2 | Surgery — X | Report to pt family — 15 | Trans-port — 5 | Hand off — 5

Anesthesia Team

ANP assessment — 10 | **Intake RN** AMD with pt — 11 | Trans-port — 5 | **Resident** Position & Induce — 2 | Surgery — X | Post-op note & orders — 15 | Trans-port — 5 | Hand off — 5

Nursing Team

Phase 1 — 15 | Phase 2 — 20 | Trans-port — 5 | Prep & Induce — 2 | Surgery — X | Extubate & Observe — 15 | Trans-port — 5 | Hand off — 5

Report to family — 5 | Pre-Op — 5 | Trans-port — 5 | **Circulating RN** Prep & Position — 2 | Surgery — X | Emergence — 15 | Trans-port — 5 | Hand off — 5 | Report to family — 5

Staff standardized work

PACU RN Hand off — 5 | Phase 1 — 15 | Phase 2 — 64 | Trans-port — 10 | Pt Care — Y | Dis-charge — 30 | **In Pt. RN**

Tech Team

Setup — 15 | **Anes Tech** Setup & Drape — 5 | **Surgical Tech** Setup & Drape — 2 | Surgery — X | Drapes down, clean, inventory — 20 | Clean up — 10 | Decontam, Decontam — 20 | **SPD Tech**

Basic Setup — 7 | Complex Setup — 5

INDEX

Capacity and Demand Planning: 181, 182, 184
Central line-associated blood stream infection (CLABSI): 97
Clinical Microsystems (see Local improvement teams)
Clinical Outcomes: 23
Coaching: 94, 99
Continuous Improvement: 41, 46, 49, 56, 88, 214, 218
Continuous Improvement Bicycle: 112
Continuous Improvement Team: 108
Corporate needs: 87, 98
Costs:
> Avoidance: 74, 75
> Benefits: 74, 75
> Healthcare: 21, 22
> Obsolescence: 75
> Reduction: 74, 75, 88

Countermeasure: 67, 68, 104, 109, 110
Create Stability: 63
Cross-training matrix: 135, 136
Cross-train: 35, 134, 135
Current State: 70, 116-119
Culture:
> Physician: 99-103
> Level 2: 137

Customer: 29, 34, 35, 41, 62, 80, 81, 100, 101
Cycle Time: 191-199, 202, 203, 211, 222, 223

D

Daily Management and People Development: 60, 65, 66
Daily Management System (DMS): 65, 204
Defects: 55, 90, 97, 106, 215
Demand: 13-15, 52-54, 63, 155-185, 229
Deming, W. Edwards: 104

P

Pacemaker: 159

Patient alignment / flow (see Value Stream)

Patient Experience: 23, 26, 29, 43, 72, 73

PDCA (see Plan do check adjust)

People Development: 5, 35, 60, 62, 65,

Perfect Quality: 13, 55, 221

Performance Improvement (PI) team: 108, 228

Physician Culture (see Culture)

Physician Engagement (see Engagement)

Plan do check adjust (PDCA) cycle: 18, 49-51, 102-104, 112, 219

Point Improvement: 85

Poka yoke: 215-216, 220-221

Price: 87, 88

Problem solving: 35, 67, 68, 102- 104, 109-112, 224

Process Stop: 17, 64, 67, 188-190, 199, 219, 220

Production Control (see Workflow control)

Profit: 87-89

Profit equation: 88

Pull: 159, 160

Push production: 159, 160

Q

Quality: 13, 14, 21-25, 55, 56, 60, 65, 73, 74, 157, 188, 219

Quality First: 60, 65

Quality Gate: 126, 198

Quick hits: 146

R

Red dotted line: 65

Reliable Method(s): 125, 190

Respect For Humanity: 221

Revenue: 74, 87, 88
Root cause (Problem solving): 91, 102-104, 109, 110
Rother, Mike: 5
Run ratio: 212, 213, 218, 223

S

Safety: 13, 14, 25, 73, 110
Sensei: 108, 114, 115, 228
Shared Values: 79, 82
Sharek, Paul: 111
Shift Length: 157, 179
Shook, John: 110
Silos (Siloed flow): 16, 43-45, 80, 82, 105, 106
Sirolli, Ernesto: 71
Smoothing (see Leveling demand)
Source verification: 215, 216
Stable Operating System: 32
Stability: 16, 56, 60, 63, 121, 228
Staff: 29-31, 84, 85, 98, 134, 188, 190, 194
Staff Experience: 21-24
Standardized work: 17, 98, 106, 107, 133, 145, 190, 196, 201
Successive Check: 215
Supplies: 56, 121, 130
Swim lanes: 196

T

Takt Environment: 64, 187, 190
Takt, Takt Time: 17, 63, 158, 161, 193,
Team Leader: 200-204, 230
Three actuals rule: 42, 142, 91
Three P (3P): 224

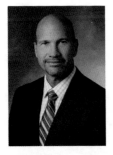

Craig T. Albanese, M.D., M.B.A., is vice president of quality and performance improvement at Stanford Children's Health. In this role, he is responsible for overseeing the children hospital's lean and quality transformations. By bringing the hospital's center for quality and clinical effectiveness and the performance improvement department under one leadership structure, Craig and his team are working to create the highest value care for the patients and hospital staff, who stand to benefit from the hospital's lean journey. Craig is also a pediatric general surgeon and professor of surgery, and he holds the John A. and Cynthia Fry Gunn Directorship of Surgical Services at Lucile Packard Children's Hospital. He and his wife reside in Northern California.

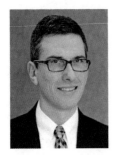

Darin Aaby, M.S., is the executive director of JWA Consulting and has been a practitioner and consultant on lean transformation for over twenty years. Currently he is focused on implementing the tenets of advanced lean in healthcare settings. Previously, he was senior lean sensei of the Worldwide Amazon Customer Excellence Systems, where he and his team of lean experts were responsible for complete lean transformations of their fulfillment center operations. Prior to his Amazon role, Darin had positions of increasing responsibility at Genie/Terex, where he served as lean transformation director for their operations worldwide. Darin has studied at Toyota domestically and in Japan. He holds a B.S. and an M.S. in mechanical engineering. He and his wife reside in the Seattle area.

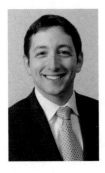

Terry Platchek, M.D., is the medical director for performance improvement at Stanford Children's Health as well as the fellowship director of Stanford University's Clinical Excellence Research Center. He is a clinical assistant professor of pediatrics and internal medicine at the Stanford University School of Medicine. Terry's career focuses on using lean to improve quality, safety, cost, appropriateness, and service in healthcare delivery. He is specifically interested in the education and engagement of physicians in improving healthcare delivery systems and the development of innovative models for delivering higher value healthcare. Terry practices medicine as a pediatric hospitalist. He and his fiancée reside in Northern California.

The three authors have worked together implementing advanced lean at Stanford Children's Health for the past three years. This book reflects that experience, including extensive collaboration with the hospital's performance and quality improvement departments and the JWA Consulting staff.

52094911R00153

Made in the USA
Charleston, SC
05 February 2016